How To Live Pure In An Impure World

A Radical Fight Against Temptation

Dan Kapenga

Farabee Publishing
Arizona

This book is a true journey of faith.

How To Live Pure In An Impure World: A Radical Fight Against Temptation

Farabee Publishing
P O Box 322
Chandler, Arizona 85244

ISBN: 978-1-68418-040-0
Library of Congress Control Number 2016961149

Book Cover designed by: Akivda M

Testimonials

Guys, you were born to win. God made you that way. He made you to make an eternal difference with your life. But there is a very real Enemy who tries to tear you down and keep you from experiencing the potential you have inside you. Too many men I know are not experiencing all God has for them because of a mind that's been tainted by Porn. But you can LIVE FREE of that! Dan Kapenga, in "How to Live Pure in an Impure World" will show you how. It'll help you "stand strong in all the will of God, mature and fully assured." Walk away from shame and defeat and into a life of freedom. This book, will provide the path!

Rev. Chris Conrad
District Superintendent
West Michigan District – Wesleyan Church

I've had the privilege of ministering with Dan for a few years now. He's the real deal. This book details Dan's journey of breaking free from lust. If you struggle in this area, you will benefit from candid but encouraging way Dan leads you along the path to freedom.

Craig Rees
Senior Pastor
Central Wesleyan Church

Introduction

Caution! Before you start reading this introduction I want to boldly state that if you currently are addicted to some sort of sexual immorality please keep reading.

I am Dan Kapenga, and I have some exciting news to share with you.

≈≈≈≈≈≈≈

I believe there is incredible hope and opportunity no matter where you are in your life. Please make a commitment to read all the way to the end.

God has given us a voice. God has given us the ability to choose which path we want in life.

≈≈≈≈≈≈≈

When I was in fifth grade an image on a simple piece of paper changed my life. The image that was burned into my naïve, innocent mind, satan used to try to dig a hole in my life over the next twenty years.

How to Live Pure in an Impure World is based on standing up against the evil of the sexual impurity of this world.

In the Old Testament, God burned an entire city and thousands of people for this same evil.

I have a wife Amanda, my ten year-old-son Malachi, a seven-year-old daughter Korrayah, and my daughter Kreana is 3 years old. I plead with God every day to help me better equip them for this world.

They are going to make choices I do not agree with and they are going to make many mistakes on their journey. Twenty years ago, Malachi would have had access to Playboy or Hustler magazines. Today the evil of the porn world is within reach everywhere. You can get it at any time. You do not have to search; it will find you!

Do you have any questions of how to protect our children against the growing annual 51 billion-dollar porn industry? This multi-billion-dollar industry is destroying marriages, churches, families and communities.

The purpose of this book is to instruct and motivate families to stand up for sexual purity in their home and in each of our lives.

God teaches us in scripture to follow him and to be obedient to His word. These chapters are a challenge to you to take leadership in your home to lead against this evil that surrounds us.

Come along with me on this journey to learn how to better instill core values and awareness to our children. Ten or fifteen years from now, what decisions will your son or daughter make if they are put into a situation with sexual temptation? What will be their reaction?

I believe God has commanded us as parents to biblically teach our children and prepare them for these decisions they will make in the future.

My challenge to you before you get into this book:

≈≈≈≈≈≈≈

Be real with yourself. Is there sexual impurity in your own life? Is your home pure right now? Let's dive into this with an open mind and an open heart. God can use this book to transform our minds into taking action with our families and communities for this downward spiraling tirade.

Let's pray this prayer together: ***Lord, use our minds and hearts while we read this book. Help us to be real with this endless topic. Lord, bless my eyes while I read this book and use me as a lamp and leader against sexual impurity. Amen.***

1ST John 2:15
Do not love the world or anything in the world. If anyone loves the world, love for the Father is not in them.

1ST John 2:16
For everything in the world—the lust of the flesh, the lust of the eyes, and the pride of life—comes not from the Father but from the world.

1ST John 2:17
The world and its desires pass away, but whoever does the will of God lives forever.

Dedication

I dedicate this book to my wife and my family. My wife has supported me through the thorn in my side. She has been my rock and has picked me up when I have fallen. I will never forget the first time I confessed to her my weakness with pornography.

She prayed with me and supported me. I am very blessed and thankful for my wife! My family has kept me accountable and continued to pray for me. My family has always believed in me and encouraged me. This battle has been a daily, weekly battle that would have been completely lost without the support of those who love me.

I also want to dedicate this book to my accountability group. I would not be writing this if they did not back me and pray for me week after week. They have stuck by me and continued to be my brothers in Christ. They have shown me what supporting someone means.

CHAPTER 1: Radical Awareness

≈≈≈≈≈≈≈

In 1993, I was in fifth grade. I had amazing parents who taught me all about values and morals. I accepted Jesus Christ as my Lord and Savior when I was seven years old, while sitting on the couch with my mom.

I had a good group of friends and I was a good kid. On a snow day from school, my friend called me and asked me to snowmobile over to his house and hang out for the day.

About eight of us went snowmobiling through the woods being crazy and just enjoying a rare day off from school. We stopped by an old rundown shed in the middle of the woods, and my friends showed me some Playboy magazines they stole from the nearby gas station down the road.

I know this all sounds innocent and normal for a bunch of young boys to do but I looked at images, I had never seen before, on the pages of the magazine.

Those images became burned into my mind instantly and have affected decisions I made for the next fifteen years of my life.

The incident was in 1993, Twenty-four years ago. There is lust, sexual impurity and sexual sin going on in our country and in our world. Are you truly aware of the challenge we are facing today? Are you aware of the differences between porn magazines, strip clubs, and access from your cell phone, your I-pad, internet chat rooms, Facebook, Web cams, etc?

Twenty years ago, I was fifteen years old. In the community I was brought up in, I would literally have to steal a magazine or make a valiant effort to get my hands on sexual material.

Today a nine- year-old has access right at their fingertips. It is literally right in front of them. They do not have to steal anything or even go anywhere to find it. It will find them!

#1 Internet

> 9 out of 10 boys are exposed to pornography before the age of 18, and 6 out of 10 girls are exposed to pornography before the age of 18. (2015 Covenant Eyes)

The biggest difference in the last twenty years is the internet. The internet is an awesome and incredible tool that has advanced so many mind-boggling events that have positively affected the history of our nation. The internet is also wreaking havoc on marriages, families and communities.

I know we all say, 'we are aware of the damage the internet can do,' but do we understand what is at stake?

I don't think we do.

> The porn industry is worth approximately $97 billion. From the US alone, the industry generates roughly $10-12 billion every year. The porn industry makes more money than Major League Baseball, The National Football League and the NBA combined. (How Big Are They, May 24, 2010)

I was at work this week and a man came to me and told me of his addiction. It is destroying his life and his home.

I am hearing disgusting and depressing stories every week about how a marriage is ending and a husband or wife is heavily involved in a sexual escapade on the internet.

Did you know the internet is a multi-billion-dollar sex industry? If your kids went into the history bar right now on your computer, what would they see? Would they be proud of what Dad and Mom are looking at?

> About half of 15 to 17-year old's have accessed pornography on a smartphone or tablet. Jonathan Blake, "Mobile porn access 'damaging' children and teenagers," *BBC Newsbeat*, 2/11/14

Are you aware of what chat rooms are doing to children? Chat rooms are a temptation that seems far-fetched. How can a chat room lead to something bad? How can a chat room derail me into sexual sin? I do not want to sound negative, but let's be real with what is out there.

We are not even brushing the surface of how scary the internet is.

I can still picture this in my mind when I was in 8th grade in 1998. I was in biology class. We had four computers in the very back of the room. I looked behind me because I heard some giggling. Two boys in our class, who got past the firewall, were looking at porn while our teacher was lecturing.

Now as parents, we not only have to be concerned with our children surfing the internet at school, we have laptops and I-tablets. The accessibility is getting worse for all of us each day.

I know I asked this earlier, but I am going to ask it again: **"Are You Aware If Your Own Home Is Pure?"**

Is technology pulling you away from God? Are we obsessed with God as much as we are obsessed with the technology of the internet?

Here are the key questions:

* Are you aware of your surroundings?
* Are you aware of how the internet is being used in your own home?
* Have you checked to see what sites your children are viewing?

It is clear in Proverbs; God wants us to be disciplined and to seek wisdom. It frustrates and appalls me to think that this growing and disturbing sin does not wake us up. We need to wake up!

The availability of this evil (sex) is growing rapidly by the minute. Again, I say: **"WAKE UP."**

> A third of 11 to 14-year old's have watched porn on a mobile device. Jonathan Blake, "Mobile porn access 'damaging' children and teenagers," *BBC Newsbeat*, 2/11/14

Your ***challenge*** today, to be aware as a parent, will be the toughest it has ever been. If you are a teen or a college student reading this book right now, I challenge you to stand up and rebuke the temptations that surround you.

You may be sitting right now in your living room reading this book saying, ***"I already know this is a problem. Why share such negativity?"***

The reason why I share this negative information is because:

≈≈≈≈≈≈≈

I believe the* more *aware we are with this issue the more effective we can be to make a radical change for our country, our communities and our homes.

≈≈≈≈≈≈≈

I believe this problem is much larger than what we can fathom. I want to become radical with this subject for my home and for my children. The TV shows that were aired in 1996 are radically different than the TV shows aired today in the living rooms across the country.

Cell Phones (Cell Phone Trust)

Per a study by *Influence Central, Kids & Tech: The Evolution of Today's Digital Natives,* the average age of children having cell phones is ten years old. Earlier I discussed how massive this transfer of availability is to our children.

Pause and think for a second, your ten-year-old is on his cell phone and, by just the touch of his finger to a screen or a click of a button, he has access to internet porn.

Remember in 5th grade 66 percent of our children have already viewed these images.

> Sexting is now the 6th top ranked issue in the list of health concerns for U.S. children. C. S. Mott Children's Hospital (2015) *Sexting and internet safety climb top 10 list of health concerns for children across the U.S.* National Poll on Children's Health. University of Michigan [Online]

I would love to believe my children would make the right choice and do the right thing; however, I know from my own experience the world has a constant pull with the evilness of pornography.

I never imagined seeing so many young ones today with a cell phone. It truly is amazing how far we have come with technology! There are incredible things technology is doing, and I do not want to take anything away from that.

However, I do want to make you aware of the evil that comes with this technology that is corrupting our children and our homes. Look at some of these statistics, and when you look at them think of your own community and town that you live in:

Mobile Porn

* By 2017, a quarter of a billion people are expected to be accessing mobile adult content from their phones or tablets, an increase of more than 30% from 2013. (2015 Covenant Eyes)
* According to Growing Wireless, 56% of children, age 8 to 12, have a cellphone.
* 1 in 5 mobile searches are for pornography. (2015 Covenant Eyes)

I again, say as it says in our Holy Bible (**Wake up O Sleeper**). I am completely convinced that we need to be radical about life!

We need to be radical about family! We need to be radical about God! Take this information about the cell phone and be aware of the danger and the temptation these cell phones bring.

I was hunting in upper Michigan two years ago, and I was in my tree stand miles away from anyone looking at God's incredible creation before me.

There in my hip pocket was my cell phone. I had access without my Dad, my brother, my cousins, or my wife knowing what I was looking at, in the middle of the woods away from anyone. I rebuffed the temptation and did not do it, but I thought of it.

Think of the porn access we have today compared to twenty years ago: Facebook, Twitter, chat rooms, web cams, and it goes on and on. I had three men come to me, in the past six months, to confess they were in the middle of an internet chat room sex affair.

I am as naïve as it gets with this subject. Can you imagine for a second what was going through my mind? I live in a conservative Christian community, and online sex affairs are going on right around me. I have had to say to myself (**Wake up O Sleeper**).

Facebook/Twitter/Chat Rooms

It seems like every year a new, quicker and better way to communicate is invented. Social media such as Facebook, Twitter, and chat rooms are all amazing technologies we have at our fingertips to communicate. My wife has had exciting experiences using the technology of social media.

She has been able to stay connected with people she normally would never have been able to stay connected too. This technology is an extremely dangerous temptation. I caution you to be aware, of not only the positive opportunities through this technology, but also aware of the sexual affairs occurring weekly through the great technology of social media.

I have heard of divorces occurring in my own community that started with inappropriate relationships through either Facebook, Twitter or a chat room. I challenge you to put up boundaries with all this technology.

If you have an extremely hard time controlling yourself with the ease of technology, you must be aware of that weakness.

I have confessed to many of my closest family and friends my weakness. I know that I cannot handle the internet in a room all by myself. I also know that I cannot handle having inappropriate movies in my house.

I will sin if I put the temptation in front of me. I believe God wants us to be completely aware of our weaknesses. I wake up each morning asking God to help me to stay pure.

Challenge

Are you aware of your surroundings? Do you ever find yourself just going through the motions in life? Life goes by in just the snap of your finger. If you are a parent reading this book, my challenge is to be real with yourself first before you even think about challenging your children.

Are you Pure?

Are you being radical about being pure if you have a lust issue? Fight like you have never fought before! Go crazy and be radical! Get help! Get Accountability! Get a counselor!

Then be radical with your children. Be aware of what technology they are using and what access they have. These statistics are growing each day. A life verse I have that my wife and I are teaching are children is:

***Biblical Challenge**:*

Philippians 4:8
Finally, brothers and sisters, whatever is true, whatever is noble, whatever is right, whatever is pure, whatever is lovely, whatever is admirable—if anything is excellent or praiseworthy—think about such things.

I believe God commands us to strive to live pure lives. This is a life verse I want to make myself aware of in my life. I understand the argument that things change and the negative stuff that comes with technology is part of the change, but I completely disagree with it.

Are you kidding me? We need to grit our teeth and get angry about this stuff. We are talking about a verse in the Holy Bible that commands us to strive to think about pure things. Yet we continue to adjust and adapt to the change.

Please be aware of how significant the change is getting. Be aware of the significance of the word 'purity'.

pu·rity (pyoor'i tē)

noun

The quality or condition of being pure; specif.,

1. freedom from adulterating matter
2. cleanness or clearness
3. freedom from evil or sin; innocence; chastity
4. freedom from corrupting elements: said of language, style, etc.
5. freedom from mixture with white; color saturation

Origin: ME *purete* < MFr *pureté* < LL *puritas* < L *purus*, pure. Webster's Collegiate Dictionary.

(Self-Awareness)- (Check Yes or No) BE REAL!

Question	Yes	No
1. When you think of sexual purity in general are you personally pure?		
2. Do you watch movies in your home that have sexually explicit material?		
3. If someone you look up to looked at the history on your computer, would they be proud of you?		
4. Are you addicted to pornography?		
5. On a business trip in a hotel room all by yourself are you sexually pure?		
6. Do you watch television shows that have sexually impure content in them?		
7. Do you have pornographic material in your house?		
8. If you looked at your household and everyone and everything in it, would you say it is pure?		
9. What does your mind look like? Does your mind look like a pure glass of water, or does your mind look like a vacuum bag that is so full that there is dust coming out of the top?		
10. When you look at how radical the exposure of pornography has become; does this scare you?		
11. Is temptation a struggle for you?		

Radical Awareness Discussion Questions

≈ Is your home Pure?

____

____

≈ Are you Pure?

____

____

≈ Are you aware of the temptations that surround you?

____

____

≈ What are you allowing into your life that is impure?

____

____

≈ Be Real with yourself! Wake up and stop living a life that is fake! If you have an issue with sexual impurity, then admit it!

____

____

≈ Are your surroundings affecting you?

____

____

≈ Is the technology that is available affecting you?

____

____

≈ Know and admit your weakness!

____

____

≈ Ask For Help Now! (DON'T WAIT)

____

____

≈ IS GOD A PART OF YOUR LIFE?

____

____

CHAPTER 2: Radical Surrender

≈≈≈≈≈≈≈

I have been battling sexual impurity now for over 15 years. For the past 15 years, I have had thousands of temptations and thousands of decisions I had to make to be pure.

I am going to be completely Real with you.

In 2005 I was on a business trip and I was in a hotel all by myself. I called my wife and we talked on the phone. We prayed together, talked about the day and talked about life. I hung up the phone and turned on the television.

I had a choice to watch one of 45 channels and I chose to watch the movie channel. As I was sitting on the bed, my mind was spinning a thousand miles an hour trying to justify how it would be ok to watch something I should not.

I would flip from one channel to another trying to find something that was not awful but would still ignite my lustful desire.

I finally turned off the TV because I knew I was getting more and more tempted to sin. The worst place for a man to be alone is in a hotel room. I know it must seem strange to hear that, but it is the absolute truth.

I made mistakes watching shows and movies that were completely inappropriate when in that exact situation. I came to a point in my personal journey where I made a personal decision to get radical with my issue.

I have made a valiant effort to make sure I am not alone. Maybe your struggle is something completely different than mine.

> 28% of Christian men and 11% of Christian women say they were first exposed to pornography before the age of 12 (compared to 23% of non-Christian men and 24% of non-Christian women). 2014 Pornography Survey and Statistics. Proven Men Ministries. Dec. 29, 2015).

Maybe your struggle is lusting with your mind, looking at sexual content on your computer, or on your phone.

Do you know what your weakness is? What is the toughest temptation you face? What do you do with this pleasure-seeking temptation?

If you're like me, it is extremely tough to say "**no**" to a temptation when you are alone. I can tell you that at 35 years-old, I have stayed overnight at my Mom and Dad's house, just so I would not be alone.

Getting radical means to do something out of the ordinary to stay committed to purity. I continue to this day to struggle when I am alone. I always try to prepare ahead of time mentally if I know I am going to be alone.

≈≈≈≈≈≈≈

KNOW YOUR WEAKNESS!
BE REAL TO YOUR WEAKNESS!
KEEP GOING TO GOD!
DON'T GIVE UP!
GET RID OF YOUR SECRETS!!!!!

Broken (How's Your Heart)

The very first smart thing I did was to get down on my knees, just like I had a thousand times before, asking God to forgive me for my sin and to wash me clean.

This time was different. This time I was not spewing out a guilt prayer of a guilty burden from a lustful thought in my mind or something lustful.

I was throwing away every ounce of my pride and asking God to take charge of everything. I was saying to God 'I was through keeping any secrets.' I do not want any secrets anymore!

I want God to walk with me in the morning and night! I want God to see the thorn in my side for what it is and to walk with me through every inch of my struggle. This chapter is by far the most important chapter of the entire book.

Without this chapter I am convinced you would fail every time. You will not wake up one day and be free of temptation and walk away from all the temptation and evil of this world.

God is with you everywhere you go. God promises to always provide you a way out. Let's stop and meditate on total complete surrender.

In the Bible, David was a man who sought after God. David has even been labeled with a heart after God's own heart. David was a king and was blessed with title, money, and power. David praised God and followed God. David sinned and lusted after a married woman. David went from praising God for all the blessings that had been poured out on him to pleading to God.

David surrendered his entire soul to God pleading with God to help him and guide him. If you are in the midst of something small or big, or if you think nobody will ever find out so it really does not matter, it does matter.

God can take your sin and turn it into a blessing. What does your life map look like right now? Where have you been? Where are you going? I know this is very unpopular to say, but the world is pulling at a faster pace than ever before. It is imperative that we take this issue head-on. I am facing more temptations now than ever.

Die to Self

Surrendering to God means to be selfless and not selfish. Most of the men and women I talk to seem to have adjusted to lust and looking at pornography is just normal. I wanted to scream at the top of my lungs when my fingers started pressing the keys as I was writing this.

Leviticus 18: 27-28
You have heard that it was said, 'You shall not commit adultery.'
But I say to you that everyone who looks at a woman with lustful intent has already committed adultery with her in his heart.

What next?

I can still picture the day in my mind. My conscience was like a red-hot glue in my mind. I sinned and let the temptation win. I felt awful and wanted to rid my disgusting awful mind of the toxic sexual images that were just ingrained into the wave-lengths of my brain.

I had sinned after surrendering every secret, every buried rock and burden in my life to God. Surrender is not something you do one time and magically your bad habits and selfish desires disappear.

Surrender is something you work on daily, weekly, and continuously on this road map we call life.

The most draining thing in the world for me is when I have committed to be pure to God, and I am successful for a short period, but then I fail.

I know what it feels like to feel God lift me out of the pit into his arms and my selfish mind eventually becomes pulled back to the world and I sin again.

The staggering question of the day is: **What Do You Do If You Sin Again?**

God talks several times in the Bible about getting rid of the old self and getting rid of the sin in your life.

I can share with you from my own personal experience this has been the most horrific war between myself and God. I want so badly, to be perfect and never sin and never have the issue of wanting to look at something on the internet that I should not.

If you are reading this book right now and you are the only person that knows about your sin and your struggle, then you are going down a long and ugly path. Do not keep this a secret!!

My wife knows about my struggle and we continually talk about it. My Mom and Dad know about my weakness and I openly talk to them about it.

Don't let short-term pleasure take away future blessings!! Get the right people involved in your life.

You can surrender this to God, but you cannot do this without accountability in your life.

The following percentages of men say they view pornography at least several times a week:

- 18-30-year-olds, 63%
- 31-49-year-olds, 38%
- 50-68-year-olds, 25%

(Pornography Survey and Statistics. Proven Men Ministries. Dec. 29, 2015).

The Five Engagements of Surrender

1. The Pride War (Humbling Yourself)

There are 24 hours in a day. There are 1,440 minutes in a 24-hour period. Have you ever slowed down and thought about your day in terms of minutes and hours? I think it is amazing that I can be at war with myself in a 24-hour period because of my pride.

There have been several occasions in the past decade where my pride has completely influenced many more mistakes and sin with pornography. Have you ever sat in a crowded room and wondered what secrets the people around you are hiding?

About ten years ago, I realized my pride was taking control of my decisions. I realized I was making decisions based on what people would think of me.

I can still picture the moments in my mind when I disclosed my weakness and struggle with my loved ones and people that cared about me.

Not one person judged me; not one person chose not to support me. I remember when I was a teen and my Dad would ask me a question while I was watching TV. ***"Hey, Dan, are you watching a show that is honoring to God, or are you watching filth?"***

I could not imagine ever sharing with my Mother or Father, let alone my wife, that I had made mistakes with my mind and with my eyes. I can remember many moments where I would be convicted of my sin in a message at church, or a Bible verse that I read in my devotions.

Leviticus 18: 29
If your right eye causes you to sin, tear it out and throw it away. For it is better that you lose one of your members than that your whole body be thrown into hell.

Leviticus 18: 30
And if your right hand causes you to sin, cut it off and throw it away. For it is better that you lose one of your members than that your whole body go into hell.

Think about what the verses are saying. I believe it is saying that if you allow your eyes, mind, tongue, or therefore any part of your body to sin, it will affect your entire soul. It will affect your marriage, your family, your job, your entire life.

If you are at all like me and care what other people think about you, I urge you to surrender the war you are in with your own pride to God.

Do not let your pride destroy your marriage. The sin, I struggled with in my own journey, started innocently and turned into my knowing exactly what I was doing before I sinned, and still I did it.

It went from a flame on a handful of twigs that kept starting and smoking itself out to a mass of logs and leaves that were flaming out of control. I would attempt to surrender some of my pride to God and throw a portion of a glass of water on the flames after my conscience overtook me.

Then I would lose a battle with temptation, and the flame would ignite all over again. I would feel depressed and awful that I lost the war to pride all over again. I have stated before I want to be real, so let's get down to it.

Pride War Questions:

≈ Do you have a flame in your life that is out of control?

____

____

≈ What is the biggest thing causing you to hide your sin?

____

____

≈ What do you think will happen if you get rid of your secrets and pride?

____

____

≈ Does your image to your friends and this world impact your secrets and your sin?

____

____

≈ God says to fear him. Can you really be honest with yourself and say that you fear God?

____

____

Unleashing Control

The last place I wanted to go to was Las Vegas! Sin City! What happens in Vegas stays in Vegas! I meet with my accountability partners on Tuesday nights. I showed up one Tuesday night and announced to the group the details of the business trip to Las Vegas.

I explained how scared I was and how I would not be able to handle the temptations that awaited me in Vegas. I explained to one of the guys that satan would attack me any possible way he could.

My wise friend said: ***"Dan, I am going to pray for you. I know that you're going to be strong. Keep talking to God about it and surrender it to Him."***

I talked to my wife in length about the trip. I said, ***"Honey, how in the world am I going to be strong enough to withstand the temptation if there is something inappropriate on the television? I am going to be in a hotel room all by myself."***

My wife, with all the wisdom in the world said, ***"Then just don't turn the television on."*** Wow, why didn't I think of that?

> 63% of adult men have looked at pornography at least one time while at work in the past 3 months; 38% have done so more than once. 2014 Pornography Survey and Statistics. Proven Men Ministries.

I, Dan Kapenga, wanted complete control on my trip to Las Vegas. I wanted to know ahead of time I was not going to fail, and I would be strong.

You are probably sitting in your chair reading this book right now wondering what happened to me in Las Vegas. Was I strong? Was I weak? How did I handle all the temptation?

I speak with the outmost humility as I tell you of the purity journey I had in Las Vegas. I did not listen completely. I turned the TV on a couple of times to watch ESPN. I was able to make wise decisions the entire trip because of the support group I have and the upfront communication I gave ahead of time, getting other men to pray for me and talk with me about this challenge.

I have not always made my decisions in the same way. Most of the time I want control and I have caught myself thinking things like:

* I can handle this on my own.
* I am not going to have any problems struggling with this.
* I am a strong person and I have been making great decisions.
* There is no reason I should tell anyone about this.

Have you ever been guilty of maintaining complete control?

2. *Accountability*

Accountability Is The First Step To Unleashing Control.

I believe it is crucial "**who**" you surround yourself with. Jesus was the master at surrounding himself with the right people. Jesus would go to parties, and he would mingle and entertain with sinners, but the core group of people he was consistently with were strong believers in God.

Eighty to ninety percent of the time Jesus was with the disciples. The support and accountability group Jesus had was incredible. You may think I am crazy for making a comparison with the only perfect person on this earth.

I compare this because Jesus was tempted directly by Satan, and we are given example after example in scripture where Jesus had to make decisions to what direction he was going to go. I made a crucial and wise decision when I asked for support from a great core group of people I am consistently around.

I talked to my wife about it several times. I talked to two of my brothers-in-law, who hold me accountable weekly. I talked to three different people who mentor me monthly, when I asked for accountability and prayer.

The most important part of change in my own life was letting go of my **PRIDE.**

I finally took away the secret, I could not figure out how to beat it on my own. Then I let go completely, surrendered everything to God and asked for help.

Hope

Every time a famous person goes into drug rehab the media makes sure the entire world hears about it. An athlete like Michael Jordan received extremely negative media press for gambling, and every time an athlete makes a mistake you hear about it from even our local news.

I was in the airport and as I was waiting for my flight, I saw a feature-on TV about Josh Hamilton. Josh Hamilton is a superstar baseball player that has struggled with alcohol and drugs over the years.

This is a man who claims to love Christ, but has been battered by the media. They watch his every move, waiting to pounce on him the next time he makes a mistake. I believe we can all learn something great from the story of Josh Hamilton.

Josh is as real as it gets! I watched an interview of him recently, and he openly shares, to the whole world, that he has a weakness.

> 21% of Christian men and 2% of Christian women say they think they might be "addicted" to pornography or aren't sure if they are (compared to 10% of non-Christian men and 4% of non-Christian women). 2014 Pornography Survey and Statistics. Proven Men Ministries.

He shares about sacrifices, he makes daily, to push through all the temptation he faces in the world he lives in. It upsets me when people, including myself, give up on people. Josh Hamilton is leaps and bounds farther ahead than most people because he admits and knows his weakness.

He continues to be an imperfect person and still falls, but he shares about the hope he has through Jesus Christ. Josh is impacting lives and changing lives while he is working on his own life.

≈≈≈≈≈≈≈

How Bad Is Your Weakness?

God Loves You The Same No Matter How Bad The Addiction Or The Struggle!

≈≈≈≈≈≈≈

Lawrence Taylor is a Hall of Fame linebacker and has had several setbacks in his life due to sexual addictions. He said something that had an impact on me recently. He said his biggest struggle in his life has been SELF CONTROL.

> The more pornography a man watches, the more he needs to conjure images of pornography to maintain arousal, and will be more likely to ask for sexual acts with his partner and have concerns over his sexual performance and body image. Sun. A., Bridges, A., Johnson, J. & Ezzell, M. (2014) "Pornography and the Male Sexual Script: An Analysis of Consumption and Sexual Relations." *Archives of Sexual Behavior.*

≈≈≈≈≈≈≈

The Biggest Struggle In His Life Was Self Control.

≈≈≈≈≈≈≈

Wow, I have made this so difficult and Lawrence breaks this down to a simple theme: We need to have CONTROL OF THE DECISIONS we make.

3. *Pleasure vs. God*

Hollywood is shining lightning rods into our cities, communities, and homes saying, ***"Do whatever feels good! Watch whatever you want to watch!"***

Growing up, I had so many people express to me that I am a right and wrong person that does not believe in a gray area. I finally realize what that means.

Think of it as a majority of our world, cities, and communities knowing the difference between right and wrong. The majority of our world is allowing this seemingly increasing acceptance of a gray area. The world continues to pull. Let me ask you a few life-altering questions.

Right and Wrong:

≈ What are the principles you follow?

____

____

≈ Has the direction of the world softened your values and principles? (BE REAL!)

____

____

≈ Are there worldly pleasures you have put before God?

____

____

≈ Do you find yourself justifying the decisions you make without knowing it?

____

____

≈ Do you follow the Bible, or do you follow people?

____

____

I saw a headline on the news the other day that Jennifer Lopez had an extremely inappropriate sex act in her music video. Jennifer Lopez is a Hollywood figure that young girls look up to and want to be like. She is a role model in our country for thousands and thousands of our teens. You look at the cover of People magazine, and their faces are airbrushed to perfection. We look at these people as if they have something that we need.

Pleasure

I think that one of life's hardest struggles is to keep God at the core and to say "**NO**" to adjusting the way we live to what our world is saying is "**OK**."

Just the other day I heard a shocking story about a teenage boy that was taking inappropriate pictures of himself on his cell phone. The school this boy attended took his phone and called his mother. The mother's response to the school was shocking to me.

She said she wanted the phone back, because she had inappropriate pictures of herself on the phone. I know I am naïve, but did you hear what I heard? This boy was living the way he was taught to live. This boy was taught this type of sick, evil pleasure was, "**OK**."

4. *Completely Broken*

Have you ever had a day, where you went so deep into a canyon, that even if you had all the equipment and even a guide you would not be able to get out? The image that keeps coming to my mind repeatedly is from the movie, Passion of the Christ, when Jesus is taking the long walk with the cross over his shoulder.

He has the blood all over his bruised and scabbed weakened human form. He is straining every muscle and using every ounce of oxygen in his body to even take a step with the cross.

I strongly believe to heal and see significant change in anyone's life they need to be completely humbled and broken down as a person to stop tumbling and spiraling in the direction they are going.

Open Arms

Do you remember in gym class, when the gym teacher would line everybody up in the gym, and you would have to follow his or her lead and do 25 jumping jacks?

You would have put your arms way out, extend them all the way to the ground, back up reaching high above your head as high as the tiny tips of your fingers could reach.

God is extending His arms to us. He is reaching out with love to take away the pain, the guilt, and sorrow.

I shared earlier bits and pieces of my own personnel journey. I shared my adventure with lust and how poor decisions on my part became a weekly and monthly rollercoaster I would continue riding.

I would ride this rollercoaster to the top of the hill, then make smart decisions. Then I would run into temptation after temptation and make mistake after mistake. I have to make a confession to you right now.

I told you I would "**Be Real**" in the introduction, so let's Be Real with each other. I asked a well-known pastor to go out to lunch with me, to get some advice and wisdom, as I ventured into trying to make an impact with writing How to Live Pure in An Impure World Movement.

We sat down at Taco Bell, and I can still visualize in my mind the words coming from his lips, ***"Dan I think that it is great that you want to work on this ministry with sexual purity, but I want you to know that Satan is going to attack you like you have never seen before."***

I left Taco Bell that day and thought about what he said. I had no idea what that one sentence, that came from his mouth, meant. I have been attacked a hundred times more than I ever would have thought possible since I started writing this book.

I have had to be on guard more than ever and have needed support more than ever. I share this with you because it is easy to read a book and think, ***"Wow this author really has this subject completely figured out."***

I am a man that doesn't have it all figured out, but I am committed to sharing my story and to being completely real about this topic.

5. Continuous Surrender

Everyone has a different opinion and a different angle of how to attack this subject of Sexual Purity. I am most passionate about this one single opinion more than anything else I will write.

Most of the guys, I have talked to, explained their journey with this sin as like a ride on the most drastic roller-coaster you can find. When you stay strong and pure your conscience is strong and you ride your way in life to the top of the roller-coaster.

The problem is the ride just keeps going and going. You stay pure for a while and then you start to make mistakes.

Your conscience weakens the more mistakes you make, and you drive your way to the very bottom of the lowest hill on the roller-coaster.

The Book of Romans has impacted my life when it comes to continuous surrender. Romans says we should have a new mind and a new body, that you should humble yourself and put others above yourself.

Reminders

* Humble yourself before God!
* If you're confident in your mind you can beat this crazy lust drug, I urge you to.
* Keep your eyes in the Word.
* Great motivation and wisdom for sexual purity is the Book of Proverbs.
* Read Proverbs in 60 days- read each chapter for two days.

According to Psychology Today, they found that people, who didn't view any porn, had lower levels of negative communication, were more committed to the relationship, and had higher sexual satisfaction and relationship adjustment. (Peg Steep, Tech Support, July 16, 2014)

Radical Surrender Discussion Questions:

* Have you ever felt like sin was conquering your life?

____

____

* Is pride getting in the way of surrendering your sin?

____

____

* Can you imagine the freedom you will have once you surrender all your secrets to God?

____

____

* Have you told anyone you trust about your sin? I desperately challenge you to stop hiding your sin!

____

____

* What is holding you back? Be completely honest with God and yourself and be real!

____

____

CHAPTER 3: Radical Generation

≈≈≈≈≈≈≈

We live in the adjustment generation! This is a massive deal! Think about it. Do you adjust to conforming to what the world is bringing before you?

I remember when I was a young boy living with my parents in the early 90's where my Dad and Mom would not allow me and my siblings to watch the Simpson's. I remember when you rarely heard or saw sexual comments or exploitation on regular TV.

It was extremely frowned upon to even use profanity on TV, let alone sex. Eventually the Technology Age continued to revolutionize into the technology craze we have today.

We moved from strict viewing policies, on what is being distributed on our television set, to virtually allowing anything and everything. Every year we seem to keep allowing more and more evil, which is now called "acceptable." Commercials that were unacceptable twenty years ago are acceptable now.

Radical Generation: (Five Steps)

I believe it is our responsibility to be a radical generation that cares so deeply about our communities, homes and children that we can take responsibility, starting with making a stand in our own actions and decisions.

A few months ago, I was at a local mall with my wife and children. We were enjoying our time letting our two children play in the kids' park while I had a few minutes to people watch.

I could not believe what I saw. I still do not know why this is a shocker to me. Teenager after teenager that walked by me was dressed completely inappropriately.

High skirts, low tops, halter tops, thongs showing on low riding jeans. Trust me I know what you are thinking. Come on Dan, this is the 20th Century. Get with the program. Things change, time changes, people change, styles change, and cultures change.

I feel passionately that God has commanded us differently! When Moses went up to Mount Sinai to talk to God, the people lost faith. They started worshipping idols and getting engrossed in sexual immorality.

32% of teens admit to intentionally accessing nude or pornographic content online. Of these, 43% do so on a weekly basis. *(TruResearch (2012) Covenant Eyes 2015 Pornography Statistics. [Accessed 29th December 2015])*

I understand that things change with time, but I believe we still need to remember God's commands. In Chapter One we looked at awareness, and how technology has caused the most massive availability of various sorts of sexual immorality. We have a choice! We have a Voice! We have gifts that God has given each of us!

We have minds! If you are a parent reading this book, I urge you to think about your own home. I urge you to think about your own circle in your life. Right now, when you look around what do you see?

What is this generation in the world right now about? In what direction is this generation going? I can still picture it in my mind like it was yesterday when my Mom and Dad would remind me to choose carefully who I associated myself with.

They would remind me repeatedly I would have to deal with the results of the choices I made. I am thinking of those same things right now.

Sometimes I selfishly do not want my daughter or son to grow up. I am fearful of what they will see and scared to death of the decisions they will have to make.

Today, in fact, I was at work and a marketing sales rep was trying to earn my business.

He was showing me his training material, and the first thing he had on the first screen was an animated picture of a scantily-dressed women that was supposed to make his software system that much better.

It truly unsettles and shocks me about the levels we are willing to take things. Does anything go? When is enough enough?

Generation Purity Questions:

* What can you do personally to make an impact?
* Which direction is your own circle headed in?
* How badly do you want to make an impact?
* In what direction is your own community going?
* Is your community more tolerant now than it was 15 years ago?

Step 1: Self Change

The only way there will be change is if we work on ourselves first. I asked this question earlier, but I am going to ask it again: Are you Pure?

How are we going to be a generation that stands up to this evil paradigm if you are addicted or have an issue with sexual purity?

I have talked to a lot of men that say something to me like, ***"I don't have a problem. I am just a guy, and this is just something that I do."*** I am sorry if I step on toes here. That is an excuse!

Men, stop using your male hormones as an excuse! God commands us in Proverbs to be wise and to stay away from the evil trap.

Proverbs 5: 21.
For the lord sees clearly what a man does, examining every path he takes.

Proverbs 5: 22.
An evil man is held captive by his own sins; they are ropes that catch and hold him.

Proverbs 5: 23.
He will die for lack of self-control; he will be lost because of his great foolishness.

The definition of insanity is doing the same thing repeatedly and expecting different results. Looking into the mirror right now you need to make a critical decision. You need to be real with what is at stake!

The only way to make self-change with pornography is to ADMIT IT, and to SURRENDER it to God. Once you have done that then you need to ASK FOR HELP! This is where the train gets derailed.

Proverbs 9: 10
Fear of the Lord is the beginning of wisdom. Knowledge of the Holy One results in understanding.

Proverbs 9: 11
And if your right hand causes you to sin, cut it off and throw it away. For it is better that you lose one of your members than that your whole body go into hell.

This is where the pride steps in. This is where the voice inside your head says, "***It's ok. Don't worry about it. This is just something that goes on in our world.***" **STOP!** I am going to repeat myself one more time. **ASK FOR HELP!**

I went to a men's breakfast at our church a few months ago, and a speaker, we had at the time, told us something that became ingrained deeply into my mind.

Don't Let Short-Term Pleasure Take Away Future Blessings!

Think about this statement for just a second. Think about how massive this statement is. God has blessings in store for you and me.

I remember when I was on the wrestling team in high school. There was a young muscular sophomore on our team that had an incredible God-given physique. He had state champion written all over his high school career.

He could have even had a college scholarship handed to him. Temptations and choices kept coming his way. Do you want to know what happened? He chose to hang out with the wrong people.

He chose to care only about partying and nothing else. The end of his sophomore year was the last time he wrestled. I remember talking to him not long after that, and I remember hearing him say ***"Dan, I really messed up a massive opportunity."***

> 7 out of 10 (72%) 18-year-olds say, "pornography leads to unrealistic attitudes to sex" and that "pornography can have a damaging impact on young people's views of sex or relationships." (Deseret News Editorial, August 24, 2014)

The reason I share this story with you is we each face different temptations. You and I need to be radical with changing ourselves when it comes to sexual purity.

This sexual temptation is going to come day and night. I hate to say this but in the Technology Age the temptation is going to get worse, not better.

Several individuals have come up to me and ask me how to stay pure when sexual temptation is all around us. This is a terrific question and is one I have asked many times.

Self-change means you are going to commit to work on improving yourself.

Self-change means you are aware there is temptation all around you, and you are committed to doing whatever it takes to stay away from it.

The misconception is you wake up one morning and say to God and to the world that you are pure.

Self-change is WORK! I AM GOING TO SAY IT ONE MORE TIME: SELF CHANGE IS WORK.

Self-change is dedication!

Self-change is commitment!

Self-change is continued perseverance.

Self-change is getting a D on a test in school and getting up early the next morning to study even harder to get that A or B.

If you are addicted or have an issue with purity, you seriously have to realize something:

≈≈≈≈≈≈≈

A Generational Change Starts With Me And You!

≈≈≈≈≈≈≈

Hollywood is attempting to adapt and adjust our communities to change what we allow in our homes and what we will pay to see on the big screen.

In Los Angeles, a billion-dollar porn empire has changed homes, communities and people for the worse. Wow, isn't it amazing how quick things can change? How badly I want to make an impact on my home and on my community for this thorn in our country's side called sexual immorality.

My mind is spinning a thousand miles a second thinking of all the ways to help my children and my home stay pure and help others stay pure.

Step 2: Stand up

Are you more sensitive to what you say around children? Have you ever disciplined a child to protect them? Have you ever said "**No**" to a child because you want to protect them?

My eyes are always opened when I watch how sensitive children are. My son Malachi will even correct my wife and me if we say a bad word.

I have watched my son repeatedly stand up in different situations as a 10-year-old. It amazes me how sensitive he is and how quickly he will speak up if he knows there was a bad word said or if Daddy did not talk nice to Mommy.

Are you sensitive like a child, or have you conformed to this world? I highly recommend that you try to get some of that sensitivity back. I remember when I was in high school, my parents taught me to have a backbone and stand up for what is right.

I think we have lost some of that backbone and grit in this country. Are you sensitive enough to stand up when you have to and when you should? The only way this generation will change is if we stand up to what is right in God's eyes.

To stand up means to have a voice!

To stand up means to say something when it might not be the most popular thing to do but it is the right thing to do.

I am deeply concerned with the direction our sensitivity in this nation is going. Are we so scared we are going to offend someone that we cannot stand up for what is right?

Why? Martin Luther King stood up for what was right in God's eyes even though it was not popular.

Abraham Lincoln stood up for what was right consistently even though people raised up against him. It does not matter where you are at in the spectrum of this issue of sexual purity.

You could be reading this book as a pure person who does not struggle with this temptation. I applaud you, but at the same time I encourage and motivate you to do more than that. Make an impact on someone else's life! Help someone who has an issue with temptation. Let your voice be heard!

Have you ever been in a situation where you knew you should have said something, but you did not? I have had that happen to me several times. I want to be that guy who is willing to take a risk and stand up for what is right in God's eyes.

Right/Wrong (GOD'S EYES)-please do not look at these questions through your eyes and your view, look at them through God's eyes and God's view.

Question	Yes	No
1. Is it right to watch an R rated movie with your family with sexual content?		
2. Is it right to allow young teenage boys and girls to wear whatever they want including bathing suits and school clothes?		
3. Is it ok to let our teens and children have laptops and desktop computers in their rooms with no supervision?		
4. Is it ok to have no rules on what music or what movies are allowed in the house?		
5. Is it right to say nothing when you are aware of an inappropriate sexual situation going on at work?		
6. Is it ok to chat with an opposite sex through a chat room or email without your spouse knowing about it?		
7. Is it right to have satellite TV in your home with no restrictions on any channels?		
8. Is it right to go to a party where inappropriate things are going on?		
9. What does your mind look like? Does your mind look like a pure glass of water, or does your mind look like a vacuum bag that is so full that there is dust coming out of the top?		
10. Is it ok to be silent when something inappropriate is going on within your own network of friends or family?		
11. Is it ok to communicate nothing to your children about sex?		

What are you going to do? How are you going to make an impact in your home and in your community? Get RADICAL and step outside of your comfort zone!

Step 3: Tolerance

It is amazing how fast time can slip through your fingers?

It almost seems to me like the faster paced life can get the more we tolerate. Have you ever stepped back just for a glimpse of what is happening around and before you?

We are all going to be different as individuals, but what's exciting is that God makes it simple for us to follow his commands.

God declares out of the text in Romans to be obedient to him. I believe that the more we obey God the less ungodly things we will tolerate.

I am finding out, as a husband, the more I focus on serving my wife the closer we are in our marriage.

The more I focus on just me the farther we grow apart. I highly and strongly encourage you to draw a line in the sand on what you will tolerate.

A couple of years ago, there was an inappropriate sexual incident at the half-time of the Super Bowl.

I remember going to work the next day and hearing how the complaints started flaring and people around the nation were jumping up and down saying how inappropriate and wrong this was.

That was a great example of people saying that they will not tolerate certain things.

Here is the definition of Tolerance:

* ***Acceptance of different views: the acceptance of the differing views of other people, e.g. in religious or political matters, and fairness toward the people who hold these different views***
* ***Synonyms: broad mindedness, open mindedness, lenience, acceptance, forbearance, charity, patience***

I am sorry to get angry, but this makes me angry!

We look at this definition and we start justifying why it is ok for us to sin. We make excuses for why it is ok for us to allow things that are destructive to not only ourselves but to others. Let's flip this negativity about this word 'tolerance' around.

We can tolerate godly things. We can tolerate things to help us grow into stronger beings. God wants us to tolerate things that are of purity and things that will help others become more like Christ.

I was in a sales meeting one time and an individual got upset and used a rather aggressive swear word that helped voice his frustration.

A couple of managers disagreed with the use of the word and would not tolerate it.

I think again we need to choose our battles, but I believe most of the time we choose not to battle at all. We choose to tolerate everything whether it is good or bad, whether it helps or hurts someone individually or as an entire community.

This deeply concerns me that I must knowingly decide what I will or will not tolerate. This is not just an easy thing to do. God makes it clear that obeying his commands will not be easy, but we will be blessed beyond belief for it.

Effects

Our tolerance of this evil (sexual purity) effects ourselves, children, families, communities and our country.

Step out of the bubble you are in and look at your community, look at the cities near you. Look at schools and children in other states. Look at the generations that are yet to come.

What do you think it will look like ten years, or twenty- five years from now? Look at how much the world has changed in the last two and-a-half decades.

Imagine just for a second how **positively** what we decide to and not to tolerate can affect our world.

We need to jump completely out of our comfort zone and stop tolerating an uncontrolled sex offender list that is growing beyond belief. I need to get out of the comfortable box

I often like to stay in and get upset and fight for my beliefs and to be pure. If you fight to be pure, others will fight to be pure. If you stop tolerating inappropriate sexual material or TV shows and movies in your home, it will affect your children and that will affect the generations to come.

Is it that exciting? I am going to step on toes here, but I believe I need to be real.

Tolerating shows like Two and a Half Men and Desperate House Wives is, I believe, the kind of tolerance that is going on right now in this world.

We are all gravitating to what is brought before our eyes next. If it is funny, we watch it! If it entertains us, we are engulfed in it!

Just the other day I had to discipline my son. I told him the reason why I discipline him is because I love him. If my wife and I are consistent and keep disciplining our son there will be positive effects, we will see from our son.

Fifteen years ago, my brother caught me looking at a website with pornographic material. He did not tolerate it and brought it to my attention.

I called my Dad, balling, admitting my shame and guilt to him. My Dad, pastor, wife, and family have helped me strive to be sexually pure, and now I am going to fight to help others to be sexually pure.

In the movie, Brave Heart, William Wallace has such an incredible passion for freedom he convinces thousands of Scottish men to rally behind him for freedom.

William Wallace took his passion and affected generations and generations! Can you imagine what our world will look like if we just accept whatever comes our way? Can you imagine what your children will see on TV in ten years if you and I look the other way and just let the world turn into whatever it wants?

I am so passionate about purity that every bone and muscle in my body is aching for purity. I can imagine the passion of purity of one family affecting another family.

This could spiral from families to churches, and to churches to communities, and from communities to cities and beyond.

William Wallace did not give up and had indescribable struggles that we do not have to deal with today. Let's look at a list of how purity will affect our country.

Positive Effects Of A Pure Home

*Respect!

*Connection to God

*Stronger bond!

*Role model for other families

*Better decision making!

*Fun and joy in the home

*Better choice of friends!

*Less conflict

*Less secrets!

*Less worry

*More communication!

*Great Security!

*Time together

Step 4: The 24 Times 7 Home Challenge

Commit for one week to make a sacrifice for the greater benefit of your home!

Are you with me?

There are 168 hours in one week. You will be sleeping 56 hours of the week, so that leaves 112 hours left in this CHALLENGE.

≈≈≈≈≈≈≈

I Challenge You To Take A Leap Of Faith And Get Intense With Your Home For One Week.

≈≈≈≈≈≈≈

Challenge:

1. Moms and Dads - Each day you will wake up and seriously commit 10 minutes of prayer for your children.
   a. Pray over their day.
   b. Pray protection over them.
   c. Pray that God would lead you as a parent and pour wisdom over your parenting and leadership of your home.
   d. Pray against the devil.
   e. Pray that God would overwhelm your home with the Holy Spirit.

2. Take 10 minutes out of your evening and turn off the cell phones the I-pads-the computers, the televisions, the radio, any type of noise in general. No matter what the age of your children, whether they are one week old or eighteen years old, spend (noise free) time with them.

   ** Let me repeat this one more time in case you skipped over this part.

   a. Spend 10 minutes of noise-free quality time with your children no matter what their age.
   b. So, you are probably simmering these thoughts in your tenacious mind right now saying, "**I already do this, or I don't have time for that**."
   c. Make a commitment for 112 hours!!!!!

Step 5: Ten Minute Zone

Let's ask ourselves an important question: What do we do now that we have sacrificed this most precious time of ours, for this 600 second time period?

My brother recently told me that sometimes the most important thing you can do when you are trying to build a relationship is ask questions and listen to the responses.

A friend of mine has struggled with a serious addiction to pornography for over 18 years and his parents never knew anything about it. The goal here, let me remind you, is not to create a perfect home. The specific goal here is to try to lead your home and children toward Christ, and towards purity.

(10 Minute Zone Questions)

* How was your day today?
* How are your friends doing?
* What was your favorite part of your day?
* What was the toughest part of your day?
* Can I help you with your homework?
* Your grades have dipped a little in math lately, can I help?
* Is there anything that I can help you with?
* Could I make a list of things I could pray for you on?
* Could I pray for you right now?

(Zone Statement) I LOVE YOU!!!!

CHAPTER 4: Radical Self

≈≈≈≈≈≈≈

I think that one of my biggest fears that I have in life is that I am scared to death to continue to struggle and continue to fail at something that I want to beat.

Have you ever thought, to yourself, that there is no reason to try to win this battle, because it cannot be won?

I have had these thoughts a thousand times. If you think being a radical person is winning this battle within you, I am here to tell you that you are completely wrong.

For me being radical meant I became vulnerable. I surrendered my issue to God and let others support and help me.

For me, being radical meant going in front of a group of 100 youth group boys with their dads and telling them about my sin and my struggle. I told my wife I felt like I was in this big hole, but I did not have a ladder, a rope, or anything to get out. I felt like I was stuck with no way out.

I felt like everywhere I looked the temptation grew more and more and all I could see were these awful sexual images. Every TV show, every magazine, and every woman I looked at tempted my mind.

I confided in one of the pastors at my church. He did an unbelievable job of listening to me and not justifying anything I did.

I can still remember the words leaving his mouth and asking me to speak at an event at church. I would be speaking to a group of high school guys and their dads. Saying yes was the easy part.

Confiding in my pastor was the easy part. Telling him all the mistakes I made and the times where I failed God, my wife, and my family was the easy part.

The part I remember most vividly is when I walked into the choir room in the back of our sanctuary at church. I walk into the room and the very first thing I see is dad after dad sitting next to their son. The pastor asked me and a couple other guys like myself to share their struggle with this life-changing sin.

I looked out at the dads sitting next to their sons and started to share some of my journey with them. Every dad and teen in the room was focused on the words leaving my lips.

Dads from that choir room that day have been approaching me and thanking me for sharing my story now for years.

One dad in particular came up to me and said, ***"Dan, thank you for sharing your story. This has started the conversations I have needed to have with my son. I never knew how or when to approach this topic and I appreciate you sharing."***

Control

The title to this chapter is radical self for one extremely important reason. We try to control and handle everything in our lives ourselves.

If I look back at the 12 years of my marriage, the biggest thing I look back on is this very exact thing. Instead of communicating with a counselor or a pastor at the beginning of our marriage, we took the control route and kept trying to fix everything on our own. Every single time we took control, the issues would become bigger, and we would deal with them more often. It came to the point where we finally decided to let go and allow God to be involved.

Open Closet

Waking up one morning and saying to the world that you have fixed your problem and you will struggle no more is unfortunately not a reality.

What do the people that mean the most to you know about you? Does your wife know of your struggles? How can you surrender your life to God when your problem is still a secret to your family and to those who love you?

Daily Battle

Sometimes I feel the perception is that this sin is easily conquered. Stay with me as I try to further explain this perception.

Moving your family from a house in Michigan to a house in California would mean you would never see the house or the people in Michigan. Your family would live in a new house and meet new people in California.

This sin, or this issue called sexual purity, is not something you can run from or move so far away from that you will never be tempted.

I am tempted every day! I am tempted as I write this book! I urge you to work at purity daily. I woke up this morning and prayed

≈≈≈≈≈≈≈

God Help Me To Change The World Today, Lord Keep My Eyes From Evil, Help Me To Be Strong Lord, And Pour Your Strength Over Me!

≈≈≈≈≈≈≈

Tomorrow morning, I will wake up and pray with passion again! I do not mean to repeat myself, but this is not something that will disappear, or something you will just get over.

I have dreamed and wished I would never have this temptation or issue again. The reality is we have to fight with God's help every day to stay pure and to grow closer to God.

I read that 'once an addict always an addict'. Each new day is an opportunity to allow God to be in my life and help me.

God Steps

It is essential you are constantly taking steps toward God. The other day sitting across from me at Taco Bell, my Dad asked me how my walk with the Lord was.

I told my Dad I am in the Word and trying to be in the Word more and more. I had to be eight or nine years-old, and I still have memories of my Dad and brothers practicing baseball in the back yard. I can still hear my Dad's strong bold voice telling me to keep my eyes on the ball as he threw it to my brother while I stood in the backyard waiting to swing at the baseball.

Every time that I take my eyes off the Bible I stop moving forward in my walk with the Lord. Anyone reading this book right now who has struggles beyond comprehension or very minor struggles with this wicked thing we called porn, I urge you to keep your eyes on Jesus and keep your eyes in the Bible!

You set the Bible down and you are putting space between you and God. I need God so badly through each temptation and each boulder in the journey.

Surroundings

* What are you surrounding yourself with?
* What kind of music do you listen to?
* Who do you associate with throughout your day?
* Who do you look up to?
* Who is your role model?

I went to a concert recently, and this wise and talented musician said, ***"If you surround yourself with people who love God more than you it will pull you closer to God."***

Stop and think about this statement for just a second. The core you surround yourself with will make a giant impact on your life positively and negatively.

I want to share again that my upmost passion in my life is to speak out against pornography.

I want to make an impact wherever God allows me, in my life, to use my journey to impact men and women towards a purity journey in life.

One of my biggest role models in my life is Tim Tebow! You hear the name Tim Tebow and maybe you want to keep reading or maybe you want to close this book.

I bring up Tim Tebow, because he is a role model to me and he continues to motivate me in my walk with Jesus Christ.

Talk about a guy who experiences probably more temptation than you or I will probably ever face in life. I have watched well over 100 interviews with Tim Tebow, and he is very consistent with his message and with his mission.

No matter how much criticism or how much temptation he gets, he continues to pursue God. I want to repeat this again.

≈≈≈≈≈≈≈

He Continues To Pursue God, And Keeps Pursuing God.

≈≈≈≈≈≈≈

The media rips and does anything they can do to make Tim Tebow's openness on his faith such a horrible thing. I was recently listening to a radio host that said he is so turned off by Tim Tebow's openness with his religion.

Tim Tebow is representing to me and to the rest of the world that we need stand up and step up with our faith in Christ.

Radical Self Questions

≈ Who do you look up to as a role model?

____

____

≈ What is your weakness?

____

____

≈ Who knows about your weakness?

____

____

≈ Do you spend time daily in God's word?

____

____

CHAPTER 5: Radical Parenting

≈≈≈≈≈≈≈

Growing up I never imagined what joy and a privilege it would be to be a parent. I also never imagined what a responsibility and daily commitment parenting is.

* How do you parent in the world we live in today?
* How do we protect our children?
* How do we teach our children about God in this crazy, fast-paced, changing world?
* How do we stay consistent as parents?
* How do we maintain strong relationships with our children?

I shared earlier that I have three children.

I do not know where you are in your journey as a parent, but let me share with you where I am in my journey. Have you ever admitted to anyone that you are scared to death as a parent? It is scary raising a child in this world! I encourage you to invest some time into being real with yourself and your home with these parenting questions.

Parenting Questions:

≈ Do you talk to your children about sex?

____

____

≈ Do you ever ask your children tough questions about their day?

____

____

≈ Who do you want your children to learn about sex from?

____

____

≈ Is it too late in the game to talk to your children about sex and purity?

____

____

≈ What is appropriate in God's eyes for your family?

____

____

≈ What does communication look like in your home?

____

____

≈ Is your home Pure?

____

____

≈ Do you eat meals together in your home?

____

____

≈ How much time do you spend each week with your children?

____

____

≈ Do you have consistent discipline in your home?

____

____

≈ Do you pray with your children daily?

____

____

WOW!

Those are some tough and mind-boggling questions to think about. I challenge parents to invest time into answering each one of these questions for your own home.

I was asked, just recently by a group of people, to tell them what my parents did that influenced me the most in my life.

I recalled the moments in the back of my mind like they had just happened yesterday. There were times when I had to literally chase the bus down the road when I was in elementary school, because my Mom wanted to make sure she could pray with me before I left for the day.

My Mom praying with me impacted my life greatly. I think the bond she created allowed me to be able to be more open about my struggles that I went through in life. Do you have a deep bond with your children?

Pure Home Principles

1. *Time!*

Have you ever had a time in your life where you wanted something bad? You wanted it so bad you were willing to sacrifice anything and go to whatever extreme it would take to get it?

I started dating this beautiful woman who I eventually married when I was a junior in high school. It did not take long for me to figure out that this woman was a needle in a hay stack.

She was the woman of my dreams and the one I wanted to marry. I wanted with every ounce of energy in my body to marry her! I was willing to do whatever it would take to woo her off her feet!

I remember lying in bed at night just scheming up what I could do to show her how much I loved her. I opened the door for her and did every creative thing my mind could think of. I cooked her dinner one time. I drove to her house in an ice storm on a day off school just to be with her. I wrote her letter after letter and poem after poem to show my affection. I spent hours watching 'chick flicks' with her and trying to do whatever she liked best.

I mentioned before that I have three children. I desire with every bone and blood vessel in my body to have a pure home! I am willing to go to whatever extreme I have to in order to have a pure home.

We live in an evil world. Satan is attacking homes daily and hourly to prevent pure homes.

If you do not have a burning desire to have a pure home, I urge you to think about our world and to think about your children.

Think of their future and what decisions they will have to make.

Think of the direction our world is heading.

Think of the responsibility you and I have as parents in today's challenging, tenacious world.

Are you spending quality time with your children?

Have you ever looked at your life and were just shocked at how many nights out of the week that you and your family are busy until 9:00 pm at night?

Is your family so busy that you are not sure where the day went, let alone where the week or the month went?

Please do not get irritated when I say this, but you need to find ways to **slow your family down!**

Trust me, the first thought in your mind is 'times have changed; it's not like it was 50 years ago'.

You are exactly right if you are thinking that right now. I am not telling you to change the entire dynamic of your family's life. I am urging you to protect your family and find creative ways to slow down. Is your family too busy to have dinner together on a consistent basis?

I promise you that instilling a monumental thing like having **dinner together** on a consistent basis will rock your family's world. Maybe it is not realistic to have dinner together every day.

Maybe reality for your family is having dinner together at the table four times a week. The key is to make it happen. Please do not read this and do nothing about it. Still, to this day, I can tell you where I sat in my Mom and Dad's dining room every night while we had dinner together. I have three siblings, and all of us kids were involved in three sports. Trust me, my household was crazy busy! My Dad and Mom had to make critical decisions and sacrifices to keep time a priority in our home.

≈≈≈≈≈≈≈

Time Is More Important Than You Or I Will Ever Understand!

Stake Out A Specific Time For Your Child

≈≈≈≈≈≈≈

A few weeks ago, my son and I had to take a trip up north just for one night. We stopped at Arby's for supper on the way up north, and the words that came out of my four-year-old son's mouth completely blew me away!

"Dad, I love it when just you and I go up north together with nobody else."

"Daddy loves being with just you too Malachi."

I called my Dad right away, because I was so proud of what my son said to me. Quality time will impact your child's life in so many more ways than meet the eye. The decisions that your children make will be greatly impacted by the amount of time you teach them and love them.

≈≈≈≈≈≈≈

Walk The Right Way To Live, Not Preach The Right Way To Live!

≈≈≈≈≈≈≈

2. *Respect*

Do your children respect you?

Think about this question for just a second. You may be wondering how and why this would relate to a pure home. We are seeing a generation of adjustment right now. We are seeing a wave of massive change.

Families are busier than they have ever been. The number of families that sit down and have a meal together is becoming less every day. If you visit your local mall you will see teenager after teenager wearing inappropriate clothing.

What are the rules in your home? Do you have rules in your home? If your daughter comes into the kitchen to say goodbye to you before she goes out with her friends, is there a freedom where she can wear whatever she wants?

If you look around in our schools, malls, and even churches, it truly amazes me what clothing is allowed.

My daughters are a seven and three years old, and someday, lord willing, they are going to be a young 17-year-old. Are they going to respect themselves enough to dress appropriately? Will they understand what appropriate clothing is? I believe our choices as parents is a massive God given-opportunity to act.

DON'T WAIT!! Start now!

Teach your children respect. I want my daughters to know how important it is to dress appropriately.

What does God mean when he says to treat our body as a temple?

I was at a church recently, and a young mom came up to me and asked me when it would be appropriate to bring up sex and purity in her home. You should start young. Each child is different. Some children mature more quickly than others.

Remember that 65 percent of fifth grade boys have already been exposed to pornography. I personally recommend you start communicating and teaching them at a young age.

Some people are going to criticize me and say there is no way you can talk to an eight-year-old about sex and purity. I believe that God wants us to be consistent in our parenting with our children.

I believe we should start teaching them and continue to make them aware of the choices and decisions they will make in life. What are your children wearing right now?

I challenge you to build a relationship with your children first before you demand that they respect you. I challenge you to spend time with them and listen to them before you can be successful teaching them respect in the home.

I will never forget it; I can remember it like it was just yesterday. I was on the track team at my high school and we had a track meet in the afternoon.

My Dad was a detective with the police department, and his hours could be crazy sometimes. I can still hear my feet pounding against the track as I was running my heart out on the last lap of the two-mile event.

I was going around turn #3, and I had not seen my Dad in the stand during the entire event.

Here on turn #3 I could see him getting out of his car to cheer me on to the finish. This made a great impact on my relationship with my Dad.

What is your relationship like with your children? How would your child react if you asked him or her a tough question about their life? Do you think they would put up a wall or do you think they would listen to you and then respond openly back?

Can you imagine how you or I would feel if our child was dealing with some radically impure and awful sin and temptation, but they had to hide it from us and keep us at a distance?

If you have a close enough relationship with your child and are asking them the tough questions of life, I believe they will open to you.

I believe the walls in your home will come down. I have talked to many teens that feel too intimidated to talk to their parents about the temptations they are dealing with at school and in life. How badly do you want to get closer to your children? How badly do you want them to respect you and open to you?

3. *Communication*

Children are being exposed to pornography earlier and earlier in their lives. More than 50 percent of children are exposed to pornography by fifth grade. A little over a year ago, I had several people come up to me after I spoke at a Sunday school class and ask me what would be the appropriate age to talk to their children about sex.

I believe you should be communicating with your children no later than 3rd or 4th grade! Each situation and child is different. You will know your child better than anyone else and can make the best decision to know when it will be best.

In some situations, you might have to communicate at even an earlier age than third grade, and in other situations you might want to wait longer.

I just heard about a situation, in the community where I live, where junior high students were purchasing marijuana from a high school student.

Talk early! I passionately urge you to openly discuss these topics with your children early!

Earlier I mentioned some ways to engage your children by asking those questions.

In the car business, my manager would always remind me to build rapport with the customer before I asked for their business. Please do not expect to be able to bring these topics up at the dinner table tonight and have this amazing conversation.

Slow down first and earn their trust and respect. Spend time with them first and learn more and more about them. Ask lots of questions with a loving heart and you will be shocked by the results.

Reminder: Communicate early about sex! Ask questions to your children! Don't tell them, ask them with love!

4. *Priorities*

Radical Generation Discussion Questions

≈ What kind of Dad are you right now?

____

____

≈ How can you better communicate to radically impact your children?

____

____

≈ What kind of Mom are you?

____

____

≈ What steps can you take as a Mom to radically impact your children?

____

____

≈ How do you feel you can personally radically impact those around you?

____

____

CHAPTER 6: Radically Lost

≈≈≈≈≈≈≈

The light I could see through thick leaves was diminishing by the second. The thoughts were already streaming through my mind. I knew I had to get out of my tree stand and travel across the swamp down the tree line back to my uncle.

I safely crawled down my tree and headed through the swamp towards my uncle. The light on my flashlight began to flicker. It went off and I hit it a couple of times, hoping my precious flashlight would somehow turn back on.

When my flashlight did not turn back on I knew, at that second, I might be in trouble. I panicked and just started screaming for my uncle.

I screamed about six or seven times when I realized I was lost. I started walking faster though the dark swamp and the water started to get deeper.

I turned to my right and quickly paced toward what I thought was a tree line and again the water began to go over my boots.

My heart was pounding inside my chest faster and faster and I was beyond scared. I didn't know which way to turn. I didn't know where to go or what to do.

This is the feeling I have experienced numerous times with purity. I have felt I cannot win because everywhere I turn there is temptation.

It is right at the grasp of my fingertips 24 hours a day.

It is embarrassing for me to share this. I am 35 years old, and to this day have made a conscious decision to have only a few TV Stations in my home.

I am not saying having cable or a satellite dish is wrong. I have barriers and boundaries in my life to help protect me from making mistakes.

My temptations with lust are by far the most challenging to overcome when I am alone, or if I am staying overnight in a hotel by myself.

I recently finished reading the book of Acts in my devotions. God revealed a few items to me that never struck me previously.

Saul (Paul) is an extremely influential figure in the Bible. He impacted country after country and everywhere he traveled he was bold for God and spoke the truth no matter what punishment or persecution he received.

The passage that grabbed me, that I can't stop thinking about, is all before the life-altering event at the road to Damascus.

Saul (Paul) persecuted and killed Christians. He was radically lost! His sin wasn't the same as pornography, but he was both mentally and physically lost.

Paul went from killing and persecuting Christians to following God and allowing God to use him to impact the world for Christ.

I cannot help but think of the endless opportunities God has in store for all of us and all the ways God can use each one of us to make an impact on the world.

Here is a list of people our society elevate: Justin Bieber, Madonna, Britney Spears, Howard Stern, Ellen Degeneres, Michael Jackson, Floyd Maywether, and Angelina Jolie.

> 11,000 Adult Films are released yearly. And the annual Adult Film revenues are $18.3 Billion. (Statistic Brain Research Institute, March 1, 2016)

We look at these individuals like they have something we want or like they are invisible no matter what they do in their personal lives.

Justin Bieber – hundreds of thousands of teenage women and girls around the world follow him in his musical career. What is his legacy? What is his influence?

Madonna has sold millions of albums, and millions of people have watched her in movies. She has influenced millions of people. What is her legacy? What is her influence?

Howard Stern – signed a 100 million dollar contract to have millions of people listen to him on the radio. What is his legacy? What is his influence?

Ellen DeGeneres has influenced millions of people in the world. What is her legacy? What is her influence?

David was a man after God's own heart. David made an incredible impact on so many people. God used David and loved David through his sin. David sinned and lusted over a married woman and then went a step further to kill her husband.

Then in Psalm 51, David cries out to God. He confesses his sin. What is David's legacy? What is his influence?

Moses was a man God used to free the Israelites and is one of the most liberating movements in the Bible.

Moses committed murder and made many mistakes in his journey. What is Moses's legacy? What is his influence?

Paul/Saul persecuted Christians! Saul murdered Christians! God takes a man that looked to destroy Christians and uses him to influence thousands and thousands of people. What is Paul's legacy? What is his influence?

Each one of us like David, Moses, and Paul have a journey we live and have an opportunity to make an impact on the world and the legacy we leave. Pornography and sin in general continues to be softened and more and more invisible in the eyes of the public.

Journey

Personally, I have been on both sides of each spectrum. I had times where I was confident, I knew exactly what to do no matter what temptation or life situation, and I felt great making that decision.

I rode the emotional roller coaster to the top of the giant hill and felt like I would just keep rising further and further up the hill. You hear of these amazing people that hit rock bottom and then completely change their lives, turned everything over to God, climbed back up the elevator in life, and were overwhelmingly blessed.

The thing that I keep forgetting when I hear these awesome stories is that you need to peel the onion back to see the greatness and life-changing purpose behind the surface.

When you finally peel back the onion you find everyone had to surrender their battle each day to God. It wasn't one giant leap back up the mountain, but baby crawling each day with God's grace and love.

I was probably 13 years old and we had a guest come and speak at our youth group, on a Wednesday night, and give his testimony. It was truly a life-altering story.

The one thing the speaker said that totally affected me was his confession of having to give everything he had every day to allow God to work in his life and help him.

Have you ever heard the saying "this too shall pass?" Temptation, sin, and the evil that surrounds us is not just going to fade away. You and I need to make an aggressive decision to keep the things out of our life that are influencing the decision to sin.

Every one of us wakes up each morning and decides to follow and be obedient to God or to live life our own way.

What does it look like to be obedient? What does it look like to be real?

Baby Steps

Every day is a new opportunity for me to live pure for God. Every day is another opportunity to make the right decisions. You can't make a giant leap to be pure until you make a small step. The very first baby step you need to make is to expose your sin.

Exposing your sin will allow God and accountability to enter your life. Starting with this step is extremely important. My Dad has reminded me, since I was in high school, I had to make it a priority to keep God number one in my life.

Number one in my work life, number one in my personal life and number one in my marriage.

Mental Block- Just recently I was in my first auto accident. I was sitting in my vehicle completely clueless to my surroundings. All I could think of was that I was alive and I wondered about the condition of the people in the other vehicle.

The ambulance came, and the paramedic immediately wanted me to go to the hospital to get checked out. I had pain in my neck and in my back. I told the paramedic "**no**" I would be fine.

The paramedic had me sign a form. He double-checked with me and recommended I get checked out to make sure everything was clear with my back and my neck.

I was stubborn and didn't want the help. I wanted to just say that 'I was fine, and I didn't need to be checked out'. I mentally blocked out help and support after the incident because 'I was fine, and I don't need the help.'

I cannot do it on my own. You and I both will fall off the cliff every time if we don't accept and take the support from others.

You can't fight through this challenge without the support and help from your community, your church, and your family and friends.

I dedicated this book to my wife, and I can tell you that she is the last person I wanted support and help from. I wanted to hide and keep my problem from her.

I wanted to do everything I could from sitting down and discussing my latest failure on the internet and my latest sexual temptation I had in my mind.

Once I was finally able to confess my sin and my struggle to my wife I saw a major uplift and impact in my marriage and in my personal life.

Satan's Lies

James 4:7
Resist the devil and he will flee from you.

It amazes me every moment to see how satan is working like a rapid speed of light! He is filling the world with lies and false hope. I was at a restaurant the other day talking to a friend about life. We both were amazed at how quickly your life can change direction.

One moment you're close to God, and then you blink your eyes and Satan has deceived you into living a life that you know is wrong. You wake up one morning and you feel alive, and you wake up the next morning and you can't believe what has happened in your life.

The most common theme that resonates in my inner core of my brain when it comes to Satan's lies is JUSTIFICATION.

The world continues daily in our social-crazed media world to tell us it is ok and tries to motivate us to believe it is ok.

Isaiah 59:1
Surely the arm of the Lord is not too short to save, nor his ear too dull to hear.

The state laws are changing and making it seem like it is ok. The definition of marriage is changing in our country and our world. Things that were unacceptable and frowned upon 20 years ago are now acceptable in the public eye.

Miley Cyrus just recently made comments that the world is now ok and it is acceptable with women wearing barely anything and showing cleavage.

Is this where we are? Is this the example of how drastically and quickly sin is becoming acceptable?

I heard someone say the other day these changes are just part of the world and there isn't anything we can do to change it.

* Do not believe the lies of the world!
* Do not live the way other people want you to live!
* Do not live trying to find reasons why it is ok to live the way you live!
* Do not try to run from God!
* Do not listen to the wrong people!

What is the Prophet Isaiah saying? I believe the verses below are passionate and carry great wisdom. As long as you continue down the path of darkness and sin you will continue moving into that direction. God is reaching out his loving hand trying to pick you up out of the canyon and all you need to do is to let him.

≈≈≈≈≈≈≈

Isaiah 59: 3-11

> 3 ***For your hands are stained with blood, your fingers with guilt. Your lips have spoken falsely, and your tongue mutters wicked things.***
>
> 4 ***No one calls for justice; no one pleads a case with integrity. They rely on empty arguments, they utter lies; they conceive trouble and give birth to evil.***
>
> 5 ***They hatch the eggs of vipers and spin a spider's web. Whoever eats their eggs will die, and when one is broken, an adder is hatched.***

[6] Their cobwebs are useless for clothing; they cannot cover themselves with what they make. Their deeds are evil deeds, and acts of violence are in their hands.

[7] Their feet rush into sin; they are swift to shed innocent blood. They pursue evil schemes; acts of violence mark their ways.

[8] The way of peace they do not know; there is justice in their paths. They have turned them into crooked roads; no one who walks along them will know peace.

[9] So justice is far from us, and righteousness does not reach us. We look for light, but all is darkness; for brightness, but we walk in deep shadows.

[10] Like the blind we grope along the wall, feeling our way like people without eyes. At midday we stumble as if it were twilight; among the strong, we are like the dead.

[11] We all growl like bears; we moan mournfully like doves. We look for justice, but find none; for deliverance, but it is far away.

≈≈≈≈≈≈≈

In the movie, The Book Of Eli, the main character is walking down a path throughout the entire movie. Every time somebody questions him he answers with the same response. He tells those that are questioning him he is heading west with his Bible in his backpack. Every time somebody tries to distract him from his journey he finds a way to continue his journey despite the temptations and distractions. Let me ask you a question and please be real with yourself:

2 Corinthians 2:11
We are not unaware of Satan's schemes.

≈ How can you become pure when you don't change anything in your life?

____

____

≈ What do you need to change to allow God in?

____

____

≈ How radical are you willing to get in your life to rid yourself of the darkness?

____

____

≈ Write down what you're willing to do to rid yourself of the darkness.

____

____

Pursuit

≈ How is your pursuit of God right now?

____

____

≈ Are you looking at God?

____

____

≈ Are you walking toward God?

____

____

≈ Are your jogging toward God, or are you running toward the world?

____

____

Be self-controlled and alert. Your enemy, the devil, prowls around like a roaring lion looking for someone to devour.

Eyes

1 Peter 5:8
Be sober-minded; be watchful. Your adversary the devil prowls around like a roaring lion, seeking someone to devour.

What are you allowing your eyes to see?

I have asked several people recently why they listen to the music they listen to. Most of the people I have talked to have said the same thing:

We Love The Beat Of The Music.

We can justify anything we want to keep doing, even when we know we shouldn't be doing it.

CHAPTER 7: Radical Accountability

≈≈≈≈≈≈≈

Who holds you accountable?

Who asks you the tough questions about your life that cause you to get uncomfortable when asked?

Have you ever tried to conquer something all by yourself?

A speaker from California, came to our church, and challenged us to surround ourselves with mentors in our lives who could coach us and encourage us on the journey in life.

You need to be persistent all year to stay accountable to God's Word. In the summer, it is tougher to meet with my accountability partners and I can tell the difference in my temptation and decision-making, when we aren't meeting regularly.

It is so crucial for me to stay consistent and to stay committed with these Bible study meetings. Sexual temptation isn't something that is going to go away!

Pornography is everywhere! Sex is everywhere! In the world we live in today, every single person needs accountability desperately.

I have a daughter, and her name is Kreana. At 23 months, she was 19.3 pounds and in the 10th percentile for her age. She was still dependent on my wife and me for everything.

At 7:15 a.m. the day started with changing her diaper and feeding her cereal for breakfast. The activities don't stop until she has lunch and goes down for a nap.

When we go to the beach or a pool with Kreana, we need to watch her every move. She loves water and has no fear. She wants to jump into the water before I am even in the pool.

Twenty-four hours a day, 7 days a week, there was an adult with Kreana. She was either with us or with Grandpa and Grandma.

She can't make decisions on her own and she needs the support of her parents until she is old enough to make them. God is with you and me 24 hours a day, 7 days a week. When you wake up on Monday morning, God is with you. When you are all alone in a hotel room, God is with you. When you feel strong and confident with your self-control, God is with you. When you feel like you can't keep your eyes or mind from sin, God is with you.

Accountability!

Three and-a-half years ago, I received a call from a friend of mine. It was 7:45 pm and I was still at work. I remember picking up the phone and hearing a faint voice on the other end that sounded like a whisper from miles away. I had to ask him to repeat himself a couple of times so I could hear him.

He said, ***"Dan can you please come over to my house? I have really messed up."*** I could hear the pain and the agony in this man's voice. I could tell he was hurt and he had hit what most people refer to as rock bottom.

I went over to his house and spent time listening and praying with him. I have been extremely blessed to watch this man from that moment grow in his walk with Christ through accountability.

Bible Study- The most consistent and impactful accountability I have had over the last nine years has been the accountability the men in the Bible study group have given me.

Nine years ago, when the Bible study first started it was challenging to get the group focused and able to get open and share.

Now nine years later we almost have to shut the valve off so we have time to study God's Word. The four men in the Bible study group with me challenge me and hold me accountable.

They ask me how I am doing with my weakness. Sometimes I have given them a very bland answer. They fire right back at me, challenging me to the core, to be open so together we can surrender our weaknesses and battles to God.

I can remember in the beginning we were more focused on having time to play each other, in Madden Football on Play Station II, than holding each other accountable and growing in our walks with Christ.

I am excited and blessed to be part of this accountability group and look forward to meeting every other Monday. I can't wait to be challenged and to challenge the others. I can't wait to hear my brother-in-law say ***"Dan, I know you are going to be traveling this week. How are you going to manage being in a hotel room by yourself?"***

This type of accountability has changed my life and has put me on a 'crawl-before-you-walk' journey to grow as a spiritual leader.

Consistency!

It is easy to be accountable for anything for a short period. One of the toughest challenges in life in any form is to be consistent.

In my marriage, I have committed several times to pray for my wife every day. Sometimes I make it a couple of days, sometimes I have made it several weeks.

This is just one example of how it can be difficult to keep consistency. We all fall short and we all sin. Throughout my entire journey with pornography my battle has been consistent discipline, and consistent accountability.

It is easy to say no to temptation for a short period, but it is much more difficult to have continuous focus and continuous discipline. My solution for this has been to have daily strict boundaries with strict accountability.

Romans 8

Romans is a powerful book in the Bible. I want to take a deep dive into Romans 8 to get a better perspective of how we need to hold each other accountable.

≈≈≈≈≈≈≈

Romans 8:9-11

> 9 ***You, however, are not in the realm of the flesh but are in the realm of the Spirit, if indeed the Spirit of God lives in you. And if anyone does not have the Spirit of Christ, they do not belong to Christ.***
>
> 10 ***But if Christ is in you, then even though your body is subject to death because of sin, the Spirit gives life because of righteousness.***
>
> 11 ***And if the Spirit of him who raised Jesus from the dead is living in you, he who raised Christ from the dead will also give life to your mortal bodies because of his Spirit who lives in you.***

≈≈≈≈≈≈≈

I have this scripture highlighted in my Bible and I have read this and meditated on this scripture repeatedly. I mentioned this before, but the fruit of the spirit that I struggle with in my life especially regarding lust is **self-control.**

I have Christ living in me and I have a personal walk with him, but God has still given me the free will to make decisions every day. Every day I wake up and there are challenges that are not going to go away or simply diminish. The direction the world is heading towards currently is **tolerance**, especially towards sex.

Accountability Definition: The fact or condition of being accountable. So, what does all this mean? How do we begin to put up the correct barriers and boundaries to shield against the technology and the temptations all around us?

Last week I was at my Father and Mother-in-law's house, and we were watching the NASCAR race. Hardees had a commercial that came on during the race, that completely shocked me. It was a hamburger commercial with a gorgeous-looking model walking around, and the TV camera focused on her chest throughout the entire commercial. This is becoming more and more tolerable around the world and in our country.

We are continuing to see our businesses use sex to sell. It is disappointing for me to continue to see this. My weakest link in my own life is self-control. I desperately need accountability in my life. I need the support of other men in my life to challenge me and to walk with me through my struggle.

CHAPTER 8: Radical Transformation Zero Tolerance

≈≈≈≈≈≈≈

I strongly define purity as a burden you will have to give to God for the rest of your life. Every time I feel like I am so strong that I will not make a mistake I am humbled by the constant temptation that surrounds us. The world is screaming an opposite voice than what God wants. Many people are going to give you a different version or opinion on what zero tolerance means.

My definition of zero tolerance:

* Zero tolerance is the willingness to work on your weakness every single day.
* Zero tolerance isn't justifying certain behaviors or sins over another.
* Zero tolerance is making whatever sacrifices necessary to keep this destructible sin out of your life.

The stronger the relationship you have with God the stronger and more visible your conscience becomes. The more you allow sin to creep into your life the weaker your conscience becomes.

When you keep sin in the dark it grows. When you put sin in the light it dies. God knows every time you sin. You can't hide from God. The only way I ever had any transformation in my struggle with lust was when I put my sin in the light.

My wife and I openly discuss it. I discuss it on a consistent basis with my accountability group. God is the transformation! God gives us the ability to change and to grow. God has to be at the center of everything. God has to be a part of any struggle you have.

My oldest daughter is extremely strong-willed. My wife and I have struggled with how to handle her when she talks back to us and when she doesn't respect us.

We read a book together by James Dobson, that encourages you, as a parent, to stay consistent with your discipline and to never give up.

My daughter is always going to have a strong spirit, but we have seen a major transformation in her since we have been more consistent with her.

I believe this relates well with the journey with sin or purity. The only way we will ever have the chance for a transformation in our decision-making is if we stay consistent with our walk with Christ.

Romans 12 talks about transformation in your life and having a new life with getting rid of the old self.

≈≈≈≈≈≈≈

Romans 12:1-3

1 *I beseech you therefore, brethren, by the mercies of God, that ye present your bodies a living sacrifice, holy, acceptable unto God, which is your reasonable service.*

2 *And be not conformed to this world: but be ye transformed by the renewing of your mind, that ye may prove what is that good, and acceptable, and perfect, will of God.*

> ***3 For I say, through the grace given unto me, to every man that is among you, not to think of himself more highly than he ought to think; but to think soberly, according as God hath dealt to every man the measure of faith.***

≈≈≈≈≈≈≈

And so, dear brothers and sisters, I plead with you to give your bodies to God. Let them be a living and holy sacrifice. When you think of what He has done for you, is this too much to ask?

Don't copy the behavior and customs of this world, but let God transform you into a new person by changing the way you think. Then you will know what God wants you to do, and you will know how good and pleasing and perfect His will is.

The only way I could reach this point in my life was to remove the dirt and the sin that I tried to hide in my life. The world will continue to pull and grind at us. The culture will continue to change and all of us individually have to make the stand and decision to following God and not the world.

CHAPTER 9: Radical Men

≈≈≈≈≈≈≈

Have you ever heard of the term "sissy"? Please don't get too offended, but I believe a lot of men in this nation are moving in that direction.

I was reading an article the other day about a movie star who suffered from depression, yet she felt that God was calling her to live out her life as an act of worship.

This movie star stood up and fought this battle against depression. She is using this thorn in her side to impact lives for Jesus.

This evil sin called pornography is going to keep tearing you away from God. What does it mean in your eyes to be a radical man?

Let me share with you my bold opinion on what the definition of a radical man is:

* A radical man is a man who loves God and is willing to take responsibility for his actions.
* A radical man is not focused on the pleasures of this world, but is focused on following God and growing closer to God.
* A radical man isn't always right and is willing to be vulnerable with any hidden sin.
* A radical man will stand up for God's Biblical values and commandments.

It is extremely frustrating to me when I see Men in leadership roles that shy away from the truth and aren't willing to stand up for God's principles and God's truth.

I challenge you right now as you are reading this to step up and stand up for the truth. My Dad just recently challenged me a few weeks ago to stand up for God's principles and reminded me that we need more people to stand for God's truth.

What is a radical man?

* A Radical Man Confesses Sin!
* A Radical Man Deals With His Weakness And Asks For Help!
* A Radical Man Surrenders Temptation, Sin, Work, Parenting, And The World To God!
* A Radical Man Leads His Home By God's Biblical Principles'.
* A Radical Man Doesn't Give Up No Matter How Difficult It Gets.
* A Radical Man Is Disciplined At Growing In His Walk With Christ.

Boundaries

Radical men have boundaries in their lives. Have you ever heard the statement, "**It is easier to Ask for forgiveness later**"? The easy way out in life is to find ways in our intelligent and skillful minds to justify and make certain decisions 'OK'.

A Radical Man Will Set Godly Boundaries!!

What is a Godly boundary? A Godly boundary is a decision that is based on God's word and God's principles

Example 1:

Bob and Tracie called my wife and I. They asked if we would be willing to go to an R-rated comedy on Saturday night.

Let's break this down:

a. My wife and I said, 'No' because we knew there were inappropriate things we should not see, and instead we suggest a couple of other appropriate movies.
b. We did not want to let Bob and Tracie down, so we decide that we are adults and we can handle the inappropriate images we should not see.
c. My wife and I decide we would go with Bob and Tracie and just close our eyes when there was an inappropriate scene.
d. I talked to my wife and together we decided if the movie got bad enough we would just let Bob and Tracie know we were leaving.

Example 2:

I had to leave for a week on a business trip and some of the other guys there invited me to go to a strip club.

Let's break this down:

a. My wife would never know because I would not tell her, and I am a man just having a great time with the guys.
b. I would just ride with the guys there, but I won't go in.
c. I can't tell the guys that asked me, 'No' because I don't want to look like a baby and have them mock me.
d. I kindly thank the guys for the invitation and tell them 'No'. If they continue asking, I would explain to them that I was going to go back to the hotel room and call my wife.

It is very easy to justify the wrong decisions. God gave us a road map with the Bible and we need to follow it.

Our World

Our world is changing, we need to wake up and take a stand for God and take a stand against evil. I saw an article in the paper regarding 72 adult men being arrested for hosting a child pornography site.

I was at our local church recently, and we had a sermon series titled the "**Get Real Series**".

One of the messages talked about how pride is one of the major reasons we do not talk about our weaknesses or our sin.

Pride can destroy our ability to confess or deal with our sins. This message was very impactful because I think the pastor was dead on. Pride is an issue for many of us.

Whether it is pornography or something different, we all struggle with sin. Then we bring it over to our closet, put it in a box, and we literally lock the box and walk away until the next struggle.

I am laughing out loud right now because the thought that has just came to my mind is so comical to me. We walk around our communities and cities daily and whenever we talk to most anyone we ask the famous question, "**How are you doing?**" 99 percent of the time the answer we get is "Great!"

The other day the same exact thing happened to me. I was at a local grocery store, and I ran into someone I hadn't seen in a while.

Right away he asked me the famous question, "**How are you doing?**" I looked at him and said, "**I'm OK. I have had a tough week. I haven't had much sleep**."

We had a real conversation together. We talked about real events and situations that happened in both of our lives.

CHAPTER 9: Radical Women

≈≈≈≈≈≈≈

Two years ago, on a beautiful summer day in Michigan I went on this annual golf outing and was extremely excited for what the day would bring. I woke up early, grabbed my golf clubs, and drove to this gorgeous golf course.

Everything was exciting all day. Number one the golf was free, and secondly the food was magnificent. One thing that frustrated me the entire day, that is still vivid in my mind, were the outfits the women were wearing on the course.

I remember both women had extremely low-cut tops, and I remember struggling to keep my mind from lusting over what these women were wearing.

I have asked my wife on several occasions why women walk around with such little clothing on. I have also asked my wife if women understand what that clothing does to a man.

If you are a woman reading this right now I challenge you to not be offended by these words, but to be inspired to dress appropriately. As a mom would you want your daughters wearing the clothing most teenagers wear in hallways of our schools and the streets of our communities?

What is a radical woman? We need to reverse the trend on what is acceptable and what is not acceptable.

MTV just had their annual awards show, and Miley Cyrus wore an outfit that basically had different shapes cut out that were covering parts of her body. The headline on the MSN Homepage read "Miley 'Cyrus wears provocative clothing."

According to the world, this behavior and a woman dressed with barely anything on is accepted.

I do not accept it and I do not even think of supporting it. It is humorous to me, when my wife and I go out on a date, even now; she will notice the inappropriate outfits and clothing woman are wearing and immediately make a comment to me, "I would never allow our daughters to wear anything like that."

My wife has a deep passion for the Lord and for the way she fights to be the best mom and wife she can in this world. It drives her crazy every time we continue to see women and even teenagers wearing clothing that is simply inappropriate.

50 years ago, you would not ever see a teenager or even a woman wearing a halter top or an extremely low cut top. Today you see it almost everywhere you look.

Honor

My son, Malachi, is 10 years old and he is at the stage in life where he still dislikes girls. He was just telling my wife and I that he does not like girls and he will never get married.

In a few years that will change drastically and he will notice, just like I still do at 35 years old.

My son will notice it in the hallways at school, in the mall, on the television shows we watch and the movies we rent.

Everything circles back to Honor. The Bible often talks about Honoring God in everything we do. Earlier we discussed that men need to step up and do the right thing.

≈≈≈≈≈≈≈

Proverbs 31-30:

30 Charm is deceptive, and beauty is fleeting; but a woman who fears the Lord is to be praised.

≈≈≈≈≈≈≈

≈ How could your clothing negatively impact you or someone else?

____

____

≈ Why is the world tolerating less clothing?

____

____

≈ What is appropriate clothing in God's eyes?

____

____

CHAPTER 10: Radical Sex

≈≈≈≈≈≈≈

Wow! Are you excited for the topic? Do you have a great sex life with your spouse? Has your sexual addiction affected your sex life with your wife?

God ordains sex to be between a married man and woman.

One of the toughest confessions I have to share with you is my struggle with sexual purity affected intimacy with my wife.

I think one thing I see now, as I look back, is a man whose image of what God wants sex to be become a completely evil and distorted image. I just recently had a Bible study and one of the guys in my Bible study shared with us that the intimacy with his wife was greatly impacted when he would look at pornography.

Reality

My wife shared with me she had figured me out when it came to the subject matter of sex. She communicated with me that I am constantly pursuing her and that my attitude towards her changes in a negative manner when we aren't intimate as often as I want.

This all ties back to the damage I caused by what I have allowed my eyes to see. I can still see the look on my wife's face the first time she questioned me about what I was looking at on the computer, and why I had chosen to look at it.

My image of sex grew into an extreme Hollywood-type view with unrealistic expectations. The more ungodly images crossed my eyes the more I expected from my wife.

All these confessions are shameful but true. My wife has been my rock through all the struggles I have had. She never gave a tolerant attitude towards my mistakes, but she challenged me and prayed with me.

Pornography

Men, it is time to get real with you! If you are looking at pornography, it is a sin. It is more dangerous than you can even imagine or even dream of.

You think you can control it; you think there is no reason to stop looking and lusting over it. You think every other guy you know is doing it so it is ok.

You think you are a guy and that guys have a sex drive so there is not anything to worry about. I have had every one of these thoughts come racing through my mind. I have made every excuse I can come up with each time I have failed.

Most guys I have talked to have done the same thing. Sex is ordained by God! Pornography is of the devil and is selfish fake pleasure that is short lived.

I am embarrassed to share that I was a complete jerk to my wife, because of what pornography did to my expectations of sex.

Do you have Godly expectations of sex, or do you have pornographic, evil, satanic expectations of sex?

I was a young guy in my early 20's that was naïve and knew very little about sex when I got married. I had images burned into my mind of awful, sinful, fake pictures.

My wife would cry sometimes when I would get frustrated because I was expecting something that I saw that was not biblical and was completely evil.

Sin's power is broken:

≈≈≈≈≈≈≈

Romans 6: 1-5

1 ***What shall we say, then? Shall we go on sinning so that grace may increase?***

2 ***By no means! We are those who have died to sin; how can we live in it any longer?***

3 ***Or don't you know that all of us who were baptized into Christ Jesus were baptized into his death?***

4 ***We were therefore buried with him through baptism into death in order that, just as Christ was raised from the dead through the glory of the Father, we too may live a new life.***

5 ***For if we have been united with him in a death like his, we will certainly also be united with him in a resurrection like his.***

≈≈≈≈≈≈≈

Well then, should we keep on sinning so that God can show us more and more kindness and forgiveness. Of course not! Since we have died to sin.

I led a Bible study a few weeks ago on intimacy, and I want to challenge you with the same challenge that I felt God laid on my heart for this Bible study.

Is Intimacy In Your Marriage Selfless Or Is It Selfish?

I shared previously that lust and pornography negatively impacted my intimacy in my marriage. One of the most damaging aspects of my sin was the selfish way I looked at sex.

The images and evil depictions in my head distorted my view. I remember my wife saying to me:

"You don't get it at all. You are always focused on your needs and on what you want. You don't want to be with me! You just want my body! You say that I am beautiful, but you don't care about anything else except being intimate with me."

I get angry with myself when I think back on those comments from my wife. She was right.

I would lust over images and pictures that weren't real and had an improper and selfish view on what intimacy should look like. What does this look like for your marriage?

God has restored this part of my marriage. God has been by my side and has loved me through my turbulence with this sin.

Is God Included In Your Intimacy?

Let me explain this question. I had a pastor once challenge me to pray with my wife before I am intimate with her. When he told me that, I thought he was crazy, and I thought that there is no way that would have a positive impact.

But involving God is vital! God has to be a part of every facet of your life. We can't pick and choose what parts we want God to be a part of. Pornography and sin has a negative impact on countless marriages in our world.

Satan destroys marriages with little wedges of sin & continuous temptation. Living pure for me meant I had to include God in everything and give him the ability to have total control.

Do You Include God?

CHAPTER 11: Radical God

≈≈≈≈≈≈≈

Have you ever seen God take a bad decision and a bad situation, and the next thing you know he is opening a door of opportunity to change lives?

I have! It brings excitement out of me to know that God can impact others through a series of bad decisions that I made. This excites and amazes me!

God loved us so much he was willing to die for our sins and our transgressions. Ever since I was a young child I had this longing that God would show a miracle or speak to me like he did in the Bible.

I can still see myself sitting in my 1988 canary-yellow Honda Prelude telling God I had the faith of a mustard seed and I believed he could make it rain at that moment just by believing and by asking God to do it.

Can you relate at all to this thought? Have you ever thought how amazing and incredible it would be to pray to God like the Israelites did and you wake up in the morning and God acts upon your request?

Through the years, I have learned that the Holy Spirit is always with me.

Radical Moments

God has taken the weakest moments in my life and used them for some of my greatest achievements.

At the age of 17, God put a Godly woman in my life that helped and supported me through the most crucial times where I struggled with lust.

In 2002, I had another section in my life where God moved at the exact moment and time that I needed him the most. I was newly married and excited about life and excited about my marriage to the love of my life.

Lust started to take a hold of me while my marriage started to head in the wrong direction and God put a Godly man, that was my manager, into my life. This manager invested hour after hour into my life.

Not only did he care about training me and helping me to become the most effective employee possible, but he cared more about striving to help me to be the best husband, and Godly man possible.

I can picture times where he asked me how I was doing with my struggle with lust, or how I was doing with my marriage. God put this man in my life. Still, to this day, this same individual sends me a text or email to check in and to let me know that he is praying for me.

The stage of my life was forever impacted by this accountability and wisdom that was injected into my life. Every individual in this world needs surrounding wisdom and direction in life. Some pastors and teachers title it a mentor or a board of directors in your life.

I have now, many years later, realized the impact these people have had in my life. Each time I have fallen or had a rough spot in any area of my life, God has provided mentors in my circle I can reach out to or they have reached out to me.

I believe most the time we fail to see when God is acting and moving in a radical way. In the moment, it is easy to see the glass half empty and see everything falling apart around you. The Holy Spirit is always with us and guiding us.

≈ When is the last time you have experienced or seen God move in this way?

____

____

≈ Write down a list of the people that God has put in your life to help support and love you through your sin or struggle.

____

____

____

____

____

____

____

CHAPTER 12: Radical Movement

≈≈≈≈≈≈≈

I challenge you to move in a direction closer to God!

I challenge you, if you know who God is but don't have a personal relationship with God, to move in a direction where you can involve the right person in your life to make that decision.

A Way Out

God woke me up recently to acknowledge that he is providing a way out of any situation at any time. Let me explain exactly what I mean.

I was on a plane heading back home from San Francisco, and I had some down time in my hotel room. I started immediately to struggle with the fight in my mind to stay pure. Anytime I am alone I have to fight through the temptations.

In this situation, in San Francisco, I was awake in the middle of the night in a hotel room and God intervened. An associate that I work with, was staying at the same hotel and missed the shuttle going to the airport. He contacted me and asked me to take him to the airport, so he wouldn't miss his flight.

This is one example where God took a moment when I was alone, with all of the temptations at my fingertips, and He intervened. Now that I can look back at my life, and at different struggles that I have had with lust, I can see where God has stepped in to provide a way out.

CHAPTER 13: Following God's Principles

≈≈≈≈≈≈≈

Psalm 119:9
How can a young person stay on the path of purity?

This one question sums up everything we need to reflect on and ask ourselves in eleven words. The rest of the psalm, the longest in the Bible, is a depiction of David laying out his soul to God of the solution to this question. David repeatedly discusses following God's principles.

≈≈≈≈≈≈≈

Psalm 119:25-31

25 I am laid low in the dust; preserve my life according to your word.

26 I gave an account of my ways and you answered me; teach me your decrees.

27 Cause me to understand the way of your precepts, that I may meditate on your wonderful deeds.

28 My soul is weary with sorrow; strengthen me according to your word.

29 Keep me from deceitful ways; be gracious to me and teach me your law.

30 I have chosen the way of faithfulness; I have set my heart on your laws.

31 I hold fast to your statutes, Lord; do not let me be put to shame.

32 I run in the path of your commands, for you have broadened my understanding

≈≈≈≈≈≈≈

This scripture is exactly what I and so many others have lived or are living. David starts out by describing his discouragement.

David then talks about God's word and his principles. When I read Psalm 119 in its entirety I get the same message and direction each time. We all fall short without God!

We all need God desperately each and every day. David couldn't fight through the temptation without God. He failed repeatedly. He failed with lusting over Bathsheba and then he acted out on that lust with Bathsheba.

It is very clear to me in this scripture that David reflected on his sin and was now focusing his effort on his relationship with God.

David lacked self-control and satan got a foothold in David's life. This one sin led to more sins.

One bad decision had so much negative impact and many consequences for David. Every time I pass a large billboard trying to lure me to an adult store I play that thought back into my mind repeatedly. ***"One bad decision can lead to many damaging decisions."***

In 2002 I was fresh out of college and had passion and drive to dominate life. First, I put together a list of goals I was going to conquer and when I was going to conquer them.

My wife and I were married in November of 2002, and in June of the same year I started a sales job at a car dealership. I can still remember telling my wife that someday I was going to make a six-figure income.

Marriage started off as a challenge, yet we were still deeply in love and loving life. One morning we finished our sales meeting at work and I went to my office to start my day. I can still visualize my index finger pushing the on button on my dell lab top. The computer seemed to be running slow, but eventually it started to come to life and instead of the home screen coming up this white background screen came up with the rest of the screen being filled with sexual pictures.

I am at work and I am freaking out!! I quickly slammed my lap top shut and unplugged it from the wall. I waited a few minutes and tried turning the computer back on by barely opening the lid so I could just see the screen.

Same results again so I unplugged the computer and put it away in the cabinet. I went home that night and had several opportunities to tell my wife what happened with a virus on my computer, but I did what David did when he looked at Bathsheba.

I tucked that common-sense decision in my closet, so only I would know about it.

This one bad decision was extremely costly in the upcoming months of my marriage and my life.

Instead of telling my wife and getting my computer fixed right away, I turned the computer on when I was not home and lusted over the images that came up on my screen.

The other bad decision I made was to justify the reason for lusting over those images. My safety net, in my mind, was that I had no control over a virus getting on my computer.

I remember getting on my hands and knees and crying out to God when I finally came to my senses with this virus on my computer. I was crying out a similar prayer that David prayed to God and I asked God to step in and take control of this situation and of this poison that kept creeping into my life.

One question I have asked myself several times, since this situation happened, is how was my walk with Christ when this temptation happened.

* How healthy was my prayer life?
* How much time was I spending in God's word studying and investing time into God?
* How much time was I spending praying with my wife?

These questions should have been asked way sooner and cause you or me to reflect and take ownership instead of justifying or strategically finding a way to deny the sin.

CHAPTER 14: Brain Damage

≈≈≈≈≈≈≈

Cigarettes damage and destroy your lungs gradually over time. There is very little harm if any when you light that match and smoke that first cigarette. The one cigarette per day becomes five, and the five becomes one pack a day.

This cycle continues and the poison from the cigarette slowly tears you apart from the inside. Most everyone I have ever spoken with that smoke, want to quit.

I know several individuals who love to smoke, but know they should quit and know they are shortening their life and damaging their body.

Porn is doing the same thing, except it is damaging and shrinking your mind. It is wreaking havoc on your brain.

God has ordained marriage and has instructed us to confine sex inside of a marriage. The very first time you look at that image or watch that R rated movie you will be stimulated and feel like you are satisfied.

Eventually that picture or image stops stimulating your brain. Eventually it isn't enough anymore and your brain is searching to satisfy the stimulation with something more. This cycle continues repeatedly.

The constant flow of these images into your mind train your brain to expect and want more. The conscious becomes weaker as the brain expects more. The R rated movie becomes the hustler magazine, and the hustler magazine becomes a full porn movie.

Researchers from the Max Planck Institute in Berlin found that part of the brain that activates when people feel motivated or rewarded, shrinks and works less efficiently: "Jama Psychiatry"

Jama Psychiatry has also linked high pornography usage to lower volume and activity in the striatum region of the brain.

This region processes rewards and motivation. In other words, the striatum is less effective when we put these images into our brain. The more images we flush into that region causes it to be numb, and unable to work the way God designed it to work.

I was extremely naive to the power that the brain has in our decision making and the thousands of thoughts that come into our mind.

Thirty-five years ago, Larry Flint & Hugh Hefner were pushing and selling magazines across our country and across our world. Today the access and the tolerance from our technology is at a level that is unprecedented and at the same time we don't realize how these images can affect our brain and our life.

I still have trouble understanding the negative impact.

In my own story, my brain has been the most challenging part to control. I had many situations where I know exactly what I am looking at, what I am doing wrong, and I was mentally not tough or strong enough to say no.

It is so frustrating and defeating when this happens. The other defeating part is the sexual thoughts I am fighting in my mind.

I have to fight against these thoughts and most importantly I have to make the right stand against the evil thoughts and give them to God.

The mind is so powerful, and it is scary how much impact the brain can have on your daily decisions and your daily thoughts.

The Beginning

Day 1: Purity Journey

(Self) Purity Journey- How to Live Pure in an Impure World

Confession: Admit that you have an issue with Sexual Impurity.

* Get down on your knees right now and talk to God. You don't have to say the right thing, just start releasing everything in you to God. Let go of your secrets and get rid of all your pride. Be real with yourself and let go of anything hidden.
* Tell somebody about your issue with Sexual Impurity. Don't just pick anyone. Make sure you seek God for wisdom on who to tell. Ask somebody that you look up to and somebody that you trust will help you and keep you accountable. Get rid of your secrets!

It is easy to find people that will tell you what you want to hear. It is more difficult to find someone who will tell you what you need to hear.

Allow that pastor or person you trust to be a part of your struggle and a part of the process to get pure.

(Parents) Purity Journey

* Pray together. Seek God as a couple for guidance and wisdom with your family
* Get out a piece of paper and start writing down the relationship building questions that should be communicated to your children.

Pray Over The Questions

I feel right now that I am pleading with God to wrap his arms tightly around me.

* I don't want to be involved in this sin anymore.
* I don't want to struggle with it anymore.
* I want to be free from it.
* I want to be free from it every single day.
* I need God to walk by my side and keep me in his path.

Write out the questions

Example Questions: (Listen!!!)

1. How was your day today?
2. Who have you been hanging out with lately?
3. Who would you say is your best friend?
4. What friends would you say are the best influence for you?
5. What friends would you say are the toughest influence?
6. What was the best thing that happened to you today?
7. What was the worst thing that happened to you today?

I promise you that your impact will be massive! Your children and my children are screaming and begging for someone to care and for someone to listen to them.

Your Notes for the Day

Day 2: Radical Awareness

* Remember if you make a mistake or fall, get up!
* We have talked through each individual chapter about being real. This isn't going to be easy and this is going to take daily motivation and daily work.
* Be part of an accountability group.

Radical Awareness Discussion Questions

1. Is your home Pure?
2. Are You Pure?
3. Are you aware of the temptations that surround you?
4. What are you allowing into your life that is impure?
5. Be Real with yourself! Wake up and stop living a life that is fake! If you have an issue with sexual impurity, then admit it!
6. Are your surroundings affecting you?
7. Is the technology that is available affecting you?
8. Know and admit your weakness!
9. Get Help Now! (DON'T WAIT)

IS GOD A PART OF YOUR LIFE?

Your Notes for the Day

Day 3: Accountability

Peter denied Jesus three times.

* Today is the day to surrender your secrets and any hidden sin. Call the individual or group of people that God has placed on your heart, so you can release all your burdens.
* The key is to have accountability.
* Do not justify or soften your sin. Just share your sin and your trouble from your heart.

Journal

1. Write down what it felt like to share your sin.
2. Pride can take away the joy and the freedom you can have in day three if you allow satan to get a foothold.
3. Question: Are you removing the (items) from your life that are part of your struggle with sin?
4. Share your journal entry with one individual that God placed on your heart.

Your Notes for the Day

Day 4: Shield of Faith

Blessed Be The Name Of The Lord!

God, you are amazing and incredible! I cannot continue this journey without you right next to me by my side.

God give me the strength today to have a pure mind, a pure body, and a pure soul. Lord provide people in my life to help me with my struggle.

* I don't know about you, but at this point the temptation is all around you and this is the time where you need to continue to surrender this weakness to God.

Question: Are you confessing your short comings, your weakness to God?

≈≈≈≈≈≈≈

Ephesians 6:16-19 (KJV)

16 ***Above all, taking the shield of faith, wherewith ye shall be able to quench all the fiery darts of the wicked.***

17 ***And take the helmet of salvation, and the sword of the Spirit, which is the word of God:***

18 Praying always with all prayer and supplication in the Spirit, and watching thereunto with all perseverance and supplication for all saints;

19 And for me, that utterance may be given unto me, that I may open my mouth boldly, to make known the mystery of the gospel.

≈≈≈≈≈≈≈

Your Notes for the Day

Day 5: Make the Right Choices

How are you feeling right this second? Where is your focus? Start your day with God!!! Get in the word!!!

A few months ago, I made a mistake at work. This incident literally brought me to my knees. I could not let go of the mistake. I could not let God take it from me and surround me with his unconditional love. I had two decisions to make.

I could admit my mistake and tell the truth, or I could lie and try to justify my mistake.

Finally, I gave it to God. He instantly took it and gave me the strength to handle the situation with integrity and to try to make a positive impact with how I handled my reactions.

≈≈≈≈≈≈≈

Galatians 6:9

9 ***Let us not become weary in doing good, for at the proper time we will reap a harvest if we do not give up.***

≈≈≈≈≈≈≈

Your Notes for the Day

Day 6: Your Legacy

* Who is your role model?
* Who is your influence?
* What is your legacy?

My role model is my Dad. I'm inspired to be more like him. Growing up I watched every move my dad made. My father walked the walk and lived with integrity.

I watched him time after time step up in tough situations. My dad is real and realizes that he makes mistakes. He is not fearful or to prideful to share his weaknesses or his mistakes.

Here is my favorite quote from my Dad.

"We are all humans that mess up. We each have our own problems and our own flaws. We are saved by the grace of God"

I know that I am an example of this personally. I make mistakes and I want to follow God's principles and his ways. Without him I am nothing. Without him I cannot fight this battle with any sin including porn.

Porn is a daily battle I will continue to fight each day. I have to surrender this battle continuously to God.

≈≈≈≈≈≈≈

1st Corinthians 6:13-14.

13 ***You say, "Food for the stomach and the stomach for food, and God will destroy them both." The body, however, is not meant for sexual immorality but for the Lord, and the Lord for the body.***

14 ***By his power God raised the Lord from the dead, and he will raise us also.***

≈≈≈≈≈≈≈

Your Notes for the Day

Day 7-8: Integrity

Focus on reading Psalm 119.

This is going to take discipline because it is a lot of reading. You need to be sacrificial and take this time to read and study God's word.

≈≈≈≈≈≈≈

Psalm 119

Happy are people of integrity, who follow the law of the Lord.

Happy are those who obey his decrees and search for him with all their hearts.

They do not compromise with evil, and they walk only in his paths.

You have charged us to keep your commandments carefully. Oh, that my actions would consistently reflect your principles! Then I will not be disgraced when I compare my life with your commands.

When I learn your righteous laws, I will thank you by living as I should! I will obey your principles. Please do not give up on me! How can a person stay pure? By obeying your word and following its rules.

≈≈≈≈≈≈≈

A few years ago, I was blessed to see an impactful illustration of how we cope in this world trying to obey God's principles.

The pastor took a large glass jar and filled it with water. He started pouring food coloring in the jar while he was speaking representing what we inject into our everyday life.

He used yellow representing work and Green, representing our family.

The last color he poured into the jar was black representing sin. Immediately once he started pouring the black color all the color and beauty that represented what was in the jar started to disappear.

It did not take much and every other representation of someone's life was overshadowed by sin. I love this illustration because it is exactly how most of us live in this world.

We do not intend to fill our lives with sin or walk down the wrong path, but in an extremely quick period we can lose complete sight of where we are on this journey with God.

≈ How does this scripture in Psalm 119 look like in your life?

____

____

____

____

≈ What changes and adjustments do you need to make to be able to be obedient in your pursuit of Jesus?

____

____

____

____

≈ What are you filling that jar with, in your life, to create the extra stress or burden you have?

____

____

____

____

Day 7 Your Notes for the Day

Day 8 Your Notes for the Day

Day 9: Confession

Isaiah 59 Sin, Confession and Redemption

Listen! The Lord is not too weak to save you, and he is not becoming deaf. He can hear you when you call. But there is a problem your sins have cut you off from God.

≈≈≈≈≈≈≈

Isaiah 59:1-2

1Surely the arm of the LORD is not too short to save, nor his ear too dull to hear.

2But your iniquities have separated you from your God; your sins have hidden his face from you, so that he will not hear.

Isaiah 59:21

21"As for me, this is my covenant with them," says the LORD. "My Spirit, who is on you, will not depart from you, and my words that I have put in your mouth will always be on your lips, on the lips of your children and on the lips of their descendants—from this time on and forever," says the LORD.

≈≈≈≈≈≈≈

Your Notes for the Day

Day 10: Stay in the Word

Your mind is weak. Everything within sight of you looks and feels like a temptation and it doesn't stop. Your mind starts to sin instead of your eyes.

God awake me,
God awake my soul.
God I praise you!
God I need you!
God I love you!
God I praise you!

A friend of mind admitted about 18 months ago he is an alcoholic. It was extremely challenging for him to get to that point. It is amazing for me, as his friend, to see how disciplined he has become, and the changes he has made to stay sober.

The other day he mentioned to me he still thinks about taking a drink of alcohol daily. Every day he has to give his thoughts and his actions to God.

He has to continue to stay in the Word and to stay strong mentally to fight these thoughts.

How disciplined are you?

In my experience the most challenging part is not only the daily actions and decisions that you make, but it is also the thoughts that come into your mind.

Your Notes for the Day

Day 11: Temptation

I recently listened to a sermon on temptation and the pastor discussed the times in the Bible where Jesus was tempted.

Sometimes I forget the fact that even though Jesus never sinned he was still tempted several times in the Bible. The key this pastor focused on was how Jesus handled the temptation.

Satan tried tempting Jesus several times and every time Jesus was tempted he made the correct decision. Jesus was in the desert for 40 days and 40 nights. He was weak, and he was tired and throughout this time satan tried attacking him by targeting his temptations.

He tried tempting Jesus with food and Jesus still stayed strong even though satan thought he had him in the perfect spot while he was weak.

Porn is all around us and the temptations come to some of us daily while others on a less frequent basis.

We have to fight through the temptations that are consistently surrounding us and we cannot do it alone. We cannot run away from being tempted, but we can control who we associate ourselves with and who is in our circle.

We can control the decisions we make every day and we can control what our eyes see. In my life God has not always been the number one priority.

My dad has reminded me often that God has to be at the center and you have to invest time into God. Every time I have said yes to temptation, it has been a time when I am not investing as much time into God.

≈≈≈≈≈≈≈

Prayer:

God, I pour out all my sins and transgressions to you!

God, I love you and I desperately want to completely get rid of this sin in my life.

Lord, I am weak, and I need you to walk by my side and to keep me from falling.

Lord, I am so thankful for your forgiveness and for your love.

≈≈≈≈≈≈≈

Your Notes for the Day

Day 12: Attitude

I recently listened to a speaker at one of our work meetings and the message left an impact on me.

He discussed several items regarding attitude, but he started his motivational speech with telling us about a personal story in his own life.

He began with your typical happily ever after life and God gave him thousands of opportunities to speak and impact literally millions of people around the world.

Then the wrinkle came 9 months ago. He had a stroke that rocked him personally, emotionally, and mentally. Following the stroke came depression and facing the fact he had to delay what he loves to do each day which was speaking motivating and impacting lives.

I looked around the room while this man was talking and he had every eye and ounce of energy in the room on him. This is a good reminder for me to look at each situation from a different lens. Attitude impacts everything we do 24 hours a day!

* What is your outlook on your life?
* What is your attitude like with your sin?

The last thing that you can do right now is to give in to the devil's schemes. The devil wants you to believe the lies and to stop fighting to do what is right.

≈≈≈≈≈≈≈

Prayer

I praise you Yahweh for allowing me to cry out to you in praise or to cry out to you in need.

Lord, help me to continue the spirit of doing what is right.

Help me to fight against this poisonous sin and to not give up.

Help me to have a positive attitude through this challenging journey that I am on.

≈≈≈≈≈≈≈

* How is your attitude?
* Is your attitude affecting your ability to fight against this sin in your life?
* How is your attitude toward God? Expand on what your attitude toward God should look like?

Your Notes for the Day

Day 13: Spiritual Discipline

≈≈≈≈≈≈≈

John 15 1-15

1 ***I am the vine, and my Father is the gardener.***

2 ***He cuts off every branch that does not bear fruit so they will produce even more.***

3 ***You have already been pruned for greater fruitfulness by the message I have given you.***

4 ***Remain in me, and I will remain in you. No branch, can bear fruit unless you remain in me.***

5 ***I am the vine; you are the branches. If you remain in me and I in you, you will bear much fruit; apart from me you can do nothing.***

6 ***If you do not remain in me, you are like a branch that is thrown away and withers; such branches are picked up, thrown into the fire and burned.***

7 ***If you remain in me and my words remain in you, ask whatever you wish, and it will be done for you.***

8 ***This is to my Father's glory, that you bear much fruit, showing yourselves to be my disciples.***

9 ***As the Father has loved me, so have I loved you. Now remain in my love.***

[10] *If you keep my commands, you will remain in my love, just as I have kept my Father's commands and remain in his love.*

[11] I have told you this so that my joy may be in you and that your joy may be complete.

[12] My command is this: *Love each other as I have loved you.*

[13] Greater love has no one than this: to lay down one's life for one's friends.

[14] You are my friends if you do what I command.

[15] I no longer call you servants, because a servant does not know his master's business. Instead, I have called you friends, for everything that I learned from my Father I have made known to you.

≈≈≈≈≈≈≈

* Are you disciplined in your spiritual walk?
* How is your balance with allowing God to be in complete control?

Your Notes for the Day

Day 14: Self Control

My wife and I took our family on a cruise last year. We surprised them and I will never forget the memories that were created from that trip.

I can still smell the aroma of the buffet food on the top deck of the cruise boat. I am sitting in the hot tub with my three children and a woman walks up to the hot tub and gets in.

She had a bathing suit on, but she barely had a bathing suit on. She was sitting next to me and I kept focusing on my kids trying to make sure that I made a good decision mentally in a tempting situation.

I also remember asking God to help me be pure in my mind in that situation. How do you fight off life situations that you can't control?

Last week I was at a Hampton Inn and the hotel receptionist was flirting with me and was wearing a low top. Again, I ask the question. How do you fight through these types of situations?

I could not prevent the situation in the hot tub, or the other situation in the hotel lobby. You and I are going to be in situations weekly that we must have self-control to make the right decisions.

We are in day 14 of this journey. The only way we will make it in this journey is to stay disciplined, in our walk with God.

I brought my Bible on the cruise ship and I read it. I spent time in the Word, and I spent time in prayer. I have many times in my life where I wasn't disciplined and therefore I didn't make the right decision when temped.

Your Notes for the Day

Day 15: Consequences

It is August 11 today and training camp is underway for 2016 NFL Football Season. Jeff Fisher is the coach of the St. Louis Rams and has been a NFL Coach for several years. Every year going into training camp Jeff Fisher has had two non-negotiable rules for his team: **Be on time and do not bring visitors into your rooms**.

One of the wide receivers made the decision to cross the rule of the coach and brought a visitor to his room. This mistake caused the St. Louis Rams to cut this Wide Receiver from the team.

The Bible talks very boldly in the book of Proverbs about rewards and consequences. This wide receiver knew the rule and broke it. He made the conscious decision to disobey the coach and disobey the team.

His consequence is going to affect his career, his income, and his life. Every day, every hour for the rest of my life God has given us principles and instructions to follow. It took me a long time to understand the consequence.

When I was a teenager I understood consequences, because my parents made it very clear on the expectation and the consequences for our household.

Your Notes for the Day

Day 16: Change a Life

God overwhelms us with grace. Does this mean we can simply give up when we fall?

Does this mean that we can justify it is acceptable to fall? One of our pastors at my church continues to challenge us to strive to be more like Christ and to continue to reach beyond ourselves.

One of the decisions we made, at the church I attend, is to plant several churches around the world to change lives for Christ. God wants to use you and me to make an impact in others.

I was at a stop light yesterday and an elderly woman was holding a sign that read:(Homeless-Need Money- God Bless)

My mind started spinning trying to justify in 5 seconds the 100 reasons why I didn't need to give that women any money.

Finally, I reached in my cup holder and grabbed some change rolled down my window and handed her the money. I have no idea what she used the money for or how it helped her. What I do know is that God cares about my heart and my actions.

≈ How can you and I be a servant to make an impact on others?

≈ What could you do with God's help to help someone else that struggles with your same sin?

≈ How could you be more consistent in your daily journey with Christ?

≈ Is the world getting in the way with your walk with Christ?

Your Notes for the Day

Day 17: New Year Resolutions vs. Life Long Resolution

At the end of 2015, I was extremely excited about my New Year resolution. I made a commitment to forego drinking pop.

You know the statistics, I am sure, however there is only a 12.3 percent success rate at people following through on their new year's resolutions.

I knew this going into my life changing commitment to stop drinking pop. In my own ego, I was already successful before I started. How hard could it be to stop drinking pop. It was way more difficult than I thought.

I only made a just over 6 weeks. I was part of the statistic of the millions of people that fail to follow through on their commitment for the new year. Day 17 of this journey is a big day. A commitment to follow God and to surrender all your sin and inequities is a lifelong resolution, and a daily, weekly, monthly and yearly journey.

I have been on this journey since I was in 5th Grade. I have had to make the conscious daily decision to give this sin and all my sins to God.

12.3 percent of the time New Year Resolutions are short term with a short-term impact on your life.

When I was in High School I re-committed my life to Christ. This commitment is a lifelong commitment. It is a commitment that God will be the authority and my savior until the day I die on this earth to live with him for eternity.

Day 17 soon will be Day 300, and quickly you will be 3 to 5 years on this journey. I mentioned earlier that I only made it about 6 weeks without pop.

My thorn in my side (porn) caused severe issues and setbacks for my life and several years ago, I made a lifelong resolution to give this sin to Christ and to surrender it to him each day of my life.

≈ What sin do you need a lifelong resolution for?

≈ What self-steps do you need to take to rid yourself of whatever evilness or ungodly addiction or sin that you are struggling with?

Your Notes for the Day

Day 18: Grace will Win

I am touching on a very controversial subject, yet I want to humbly make a couple of statements. I have had the thought in my own mind several times that I am a Christian and God will love me forever and forever.

He will forgive me 70 times 7. Everyone falls short, everyone sins, and this sin is just a part of my life. God will overwhelm me with grace and I can continue this path I have been on.

I know it is wrong and is ungodly, but it is what it is.

God is a massive God and will forgive us, yet I think many of us are being misled here just like some of the thoughts I just shared. It is very clear in the Bible there are consequences for sin. God has many gifts and treasures in store for us in heaven.

This is a very important day for you and it is paramount you fight like you have never fought before. Over the course of 35 years, of my life, we have seen a world that has changed and is becoming more and more tolerant each day.

Last week our pastor preached a sermon on the Holy Spirit.

My greatest takeaway in that message was 'some of us, in this world, are waiting for that magic moment where God is going to speak, in the volume of a large magnificent fashion, to make his vision and purpose for our life known.'

The fact is God does speak that way. God also wants us to have faith of a mustard seed, discern and listen to the Holy Spirit and to follow his will and purpose.

The dot I am trying to connect is that God wants us to do something with our sin no matter our struggle in life. Have you ever thought that God may have already spoken to you, but you didn't hear him?

I personally struggled with my sin, for a crazy length of time, before I really heard God's voice. I drowned out his voice and the Holy Spirit knocking on my heart.

Sin was winning the battle until I finally allowed God to have complete control. Now 15 years later I am trying to make an impact with the daily decisions I make and with helping others who have the same struggle I had.

≈ I boldly ask you right now what you are doing to help someone else that has the same struggle as you?

____

____

____

____

____

____

____

____

≈ How much time are you carving out of each day to invest into hearing God? Write down an action plan of how you can make this a priority of each day.

____

____

____

____

____

____

Your Notes for the Day

Day 19: Most Important Lessons

One of the most important lessons, I continue to learn in life, is that no matter how good or bad the situation you are in, God is in control.

In the last couple of weeks, I made a couple of mental errors at work. These errors cause stress, emotion, and could have been prevented if I would have slowed down the pace and cross checked my work.

I am guilty of allowing myself to take on so much in work and life I start making errors that are completely controllable.

Sin is the same way. Just think about it. We can give our sin to God and surrender it to him. Many times, we take a different path and try to control and handle our sin ourselves. Today we are going to study and look out.

≈≈≈≈≈≈≈

Ephesians 5. 1-7

1 Follow God's example, therefore, as dearly loved children

2 and walk in the way of love, just as Christ loved us and gave himself up for us as a fragrant offering and sacrifice to God.

[3] But among you there must not be even a hint of sexual immorality, or of any kind of impurity, or of greed, because these are improper for God's holy people.

[4] Nor should there be obscenity, foolish talk or coarse joking, which are out of place, but rather thanksgiving.

[5] For of this you can be sure: No immoral, impure or greedy person—such a person is an idolater—has any inheritance in the kingdom of Christ and of God.

[6] Let no one deceive you with empty words, for because of such things God's wrath comes on those who are disobedient.

[7] Therefore do not be partners with them.

≈≈≈≈≈≈≈

Every time I open God's Word I am challenged, amazed, and inspired to grow closer to him. In Ephesians, the message is direct and clear about sexual immorality. The word is also clear about many other sins as well.

I believe the simple message here is that we need to surrender any of these sins in our lives to Christ. This scripture is also extremely clear there is a consequence for sin and for following the world and not God.

Let's look at one more passage in Ephesians.

≈≈≈≈≈≈≈

Ephesians 5. 8-14

8 ***For you were once darkness, but now you are light in the Lord. Live as children of light***

9 ***(for the fruit of the light consists in all goodness, righteousness and truth)***

10 ***and find out what pleases the Lord.***

11 ***Have nothing to do with the fruitless deeds of darkness, but rather expose them.***

≈≈≈≈≈≈≈

It is shameful even to mention what the disobedient do in secret. But everything exposed by the light becomes visible- and everything that is illuminated becomes a light. Therefore, it is said:

'Wake up, sleeper,
Rise from the dead,
And Christ will shine on you"

Again, the message is clear as crystal here that we are to live in the light and expose any of the darkness in our lives. It is completely and utterly shameful to keep it hidden or to keep our sin a secret.

≈ Is there any sin in your life right now that you still are hiding? Share what the sin is and why you have been hiding it so long.

≈ We are 19 days into this Journey. How are you doing with total surrender to God with your weakness?

≈ Write a list of the individuals in your life that are helping to support you and hold you accountable.

____

____

____

____

____

____

____

____

≈ What is your action plan after this 20-day journey? What are you going to do to keep your sin exposed and to continue to surrender your sin to God?

____

____

____

____

____

____

____

Your Notes for the Day

Day 20: Challenge

Wow, it is amazing at how quickly 20 days can come and go! This is a snap shot of the daily focus and investment you need to make each day to expose all your sin and to give all of it to Christ.

I thank you for taking the time to go through this book with me and to journey through the last 20 days together. I was reminded this week it is better to slow down, than speed up in life.

Writing this book reminded me again and again I need to take this life one day at a time. Each morning I need to wake up and surrender my day and my journey to God.

The sin I battled was a 15-year struggle and I continue to give to God each day.

CHALLENGE

I want to leave you with one challenge. There are many people in this world struggling with the same sin or issue you are struggling with.

I urge you to pray to God that he would put someone in your life you could impact. I urge you to do something when God puts that person in your mind. Take a step and use the gifts God has given you to impact another life for Christ!!!!!